THE WEIGHT OF ADDICTION

TRANSFORMING ACTIVITIES & HABITS

MILTON HARRISON

© Copyright 2020 - All rights reserved.

It is not legal to reproduce, duplicate, or transmit any part of this document in either electronic means or in printed format. Recording of this publication is strictly prohibited and any storage of this document is not allowed unless with written permission from the publisher except for the use of brief quotations in a book review.

CONTENTS

Introduction   5

1. What Is Addiction?   9
2. How Addiction Happens   29
3. Understanding the Past in Order to Build a Future   42
4. A Balanced and Purposeful Life is a Sober Life   51
5. Developing New Habits   68
6. Staying Active to Move Forward   82
7. In Review   91
8. Conclusion   102

References   105

INTRODUCTION

"It does not matter how slowly you go as long as you do not stop."

— CONFUCIUS

Freedom is the greatest motivator. People have started revolutions, wars, and movements because of this universal truth. Humanity has scaled higher levels of education and knowledge in order to achieve it, for true liberation that can only be obtained through insight. Freedom has a variety of meanings to different people. This personal, individual definition depends on one's background, and the reasoning behind their desire for it.

Addiction, in itself, is a restriction of that freedom. It weighs you down and creates a vast array of difficulties preventing you from becoming the best you can be. Perhaps, in your situation, you want to be a better student and take your grades and academic priorities seriously, but you just can't seem to get it down. This is not because you have any literacy issues, and it certainly is not because you are lacking in intelligence. When you took the time to figure out why, it turned out you had an addiction to playing video games. While this may seem trivial, it is far from that; in fact, there is great importance there. You find, after doing some self-discovery, that you can hardly function without playing video games. It has begun to take a toll on other parts of your life: socializing, family, and interests in general. It is scary to admit, but the facts remain.

Maybe your personal experience is that you can't go a day without smoking. There has been justification in the past because you don't smoke a pack a day, but you just are not able to stop. Whenever you need to cope with something, you reach for a cigarette. When stress is introduced to your life, you go for a cigarette again. Recognizing this pattern is incredibly important, but it still is only a first step.

Whether your addiction is drugs, alcohol, gambling, watching pornography, exercising, or even eating, you must come to the realization that it hinders you from maximizing your potential. Addiction weighs you down.

The possibilities of a life free from the downward spirals and destruction of addiction are endless. This book and the lessons within will expose you to the benefits of living a life without the restrictions and pain that can come from the cycles of an addict. and can serve as a guide for your entire journey. A life after addiction will bring you the opportunity to have better relationships, healthy and productive hobbies, and self-fulfillment. Every step you take on your journey to a new, fresh, revitalized life is worth it. *You* are worth it.

During the course of this journey, you will learn how to alter your perspectives to regain a healthy outlook on life, and the correct images of both yourself and the life you are leading. You will be uplifted and challenged, but never judged. You have either been a victim of extreme judgement, or you have known someone who has experienced that; both are far too prevalent in the lives of those going through the recovery process. Above all, you are a good person who has realized the direction their life was headed, and mustered the strength to make a change. With that change, that life altering choice, you began a series of forward-moving steps that will gradually lead you into a life that is bright and filled with potential.

This book is for everyone who can relate to the challenging situations we just laid out. This book is for all of us who struggled, or still struggle with drugs, alcohol, gambling, shopping, eating, exercising, or whatever addiction has eaten away at both your joy and life. I can promise you that this book will provide you with the knowledge, tools, and techniques you need to overcome addiction. This set of guidelines will change the way you look at life. You will know what it is like to be empowered with the courage to take control back by casting off the shackles of addiction. If you are struggling with addiction in any way, this book provides you with a step-by-step guide on how to break free from it. You will learn activities that you can get involved in to free yourself, as well as habits that you have to break or relearn.

The information that will be covered is an in-depth guide on this type of dependence and the ways in which you can overcome it to move forward into a life of purpose. This information is not a substitute for medical attention, and neither is it a replacement for the recommended therapy or support groups deemed necessary for one's journey to a life free of addiction. If you are worried or anxious about the changes you will have to make in your life, remember that you don't have to do it all at once. You can take it slowly. In fact, it is both suggested and healthy to have a steady, healthy approach. You do not want to rush into these kinds of changes because it will most likely drain you of whatever drive you have. As long as you are consistent and committed, you will achieve your goal. You will break free of your addiction to discover a full life on the other side.

If you want to free yourself from the weight of addiction, you need to properly understand what that truly means, what the definition is in all its forms. The first step to free yourself from a life beholden to that addictive act or substance is to understand what the cause or the root is. Beginning with the first chapter, and for the remainder of our time together, you will start to unravel the pain, challenges, and depth that exist within the life you are trying to leave behind. With trust, inspired action, and your capable strength there is nothing you cannot achieve, including a life of sobriety.

1

WHAT IS ADDICTION?

A few years ago, I heard about a boy, a young man now, who lost both his parents in an unfortunate accident. He was in college when it happened. When he heard about it, this young man turned to alcohol to cope with his grief. The more time passed, the more he would use drinking to mask even more pain. He eventually developed such a strong dependency on it that he started skipping classes, stopped turning in homework, and lost the friends he had through continued isolation and drastic personality changes. As the difficulties and consequences piled up, he reached a point where he had to drop out of college. It wasn't an overnight change, but his life was overtaken at a gradual, wretched pace.

It has become far too commonplace for people to hear stories like this cautionary tale of people whose lives have taken a turn for the worse - or ended - because of addiction. Maybe you are even one of the afflicted whose lives have changed to these extreme degrees. Perhaps a similar experience followed that same steady destruction to where you have lost your job. The damages are far-reaching, spreading to relationships, your sense of autonomy, your finances but you can gain it all back. It takes work and dedication, but it can happen. *You* can make it happen but not without taking action.

Through the ages, humanity has struggled with addictions to various substances such as alcohol, cannabis, and cocaine, to name some of the better known offenders. The dissuasion from intoxication common is an occurrence across all societies in different eras. In fact, some cultures restricted the use of some substances to specific rituals or events. For the ancient Aztecs, alcohol served a ceremonial purpose and its consumption outside of such purpose was punishable by death. Even ancient philosophers and physicians recognized the possibility of addiction, as well as the dangers of substances such as alcohol or opium. Aristotle recognized the harmful effects of alcohol consumption on pregnant women and studied the side effects of alcohol withdrawal.

Addiction became an even more prominent issue upon industrialization, colonization, and globalization. As international trade became more possible, alcohol and other substances were made available for the population. In the 18th Century, Benjamin Rush, an American physicist, posited that the lack of self-control by drinkers was caused by the drink rather than the drinkers. In the 19th Century, medical journals were created for the purpose of studying addiction. This study was influenced by the opiate addiction that ravaged America and Europe. No matter the time period, the same story was being told with different characters. Each passing century saw the world grow a little smaller, a little closer together, until cultural exports were reaching places never before thought possible. While this introduced many positive aspects into the international scene, when a substance arrived that held the addictive potential as the previously mentioned examples, the results were usually a documented pattern.

In recent years, addiction has continued to move towards the forefront of both policy and public opinion, with a focus on substance abuse being the primary link to addiction. According to the World

Drug Report released by the United Nations Office on Drugs and Crime (UNODC) in 2019, about 35 million people worldwide suffer from a form substance use disorder. The report estimates the number of opioid users worldwide to be 53 million, putting the figures higher than that of the other types of drug use disorder. These figures resonate with even more impact when you consider the number of Americans that suffer from substance use disorder. The National Survey on Drug Use and Health (NSDUH) reported that 19.7 million Americans struggled with substance use disorder in 2017. Considering the exponential growth of the afflicted, every day the issue becomes more dire.

Addiction can be defined by some as the abnormal dependence of a person on an activity or a habit-forming substance to the point where abstinence from the cause of the addiction inflicts negative symptoms. Addiction is a rather complex condition. Despite its harmful and disproportionately negative consequences on the mind and body of an individual suffering from addiction, it maintains its hold on such a person. When the brain is constantly exposed to addictive stimuli such as gambling, the use of drugs, the rush or high that comes with playing video games, and a variety of other possible circumstances, it begins to crave the rewards that are associated with such activities. Addiction to substances progress from use to abuse to dependence: this is how the body comes to require the substance to function.

There isn't a switch that suddenly flips, turning someone from a non-user into a user. The process usually goes unrecognized for some time, especially when the overuse is an effective masking agent for whatever the person is trying to escape. That bond between not feeling pain - physical or emotional - begins to create that belief within the mind that without the substance or act, the pain will come flooding back. Addressing the subject of addiction is never a simple thing; in fact, when done correctly, it painstakingly reveals layers upon layers of introspection before real healing can begin. Without recognizing the many areas that impact the intensity of the addiction, you are not going to be following the best path to freedom, peace, and true remedy.

Addiction may sometimes be mistaken for misuse, especially on the topic of substance consumption. The two concepts are different, despite sharing some similarities. A person may misuse drugs by taking more than was prescribed by a qualified doctor or physician but they may not, in fact, be addicted to the drugs. In such a scenario, addiction happens when the individual cannot do without the consumption of the drugs, in an even higher quantity. Oftentimes, misuse of substances leads to addiction. The crossing of that line usually occurs when the misuse ends up "treating" another symptom: pain medication to mentally avoid dealing with financial burdens; steroids meant for inflammation used to try a back-alley way of bulking up. While the initial medication, or substance, was obtained for a health-conscious, medically-approved reason with specific instructions, the methods in which it was used created the right environment for addiction to thrive.

A person suffering from addiction may not realize what they are going through. Addiction to certain activities or substances can blur a person's sense of self-reflection. It is therefore important for one to know the common symptoms of a person struggling with addiction of any kind. By taking the time to identify both the stages of addiction as well as the underlying factors behind those stages, you are allowing yourself the chance to heal - maybe for the first time in your life.

When dealing with the surrounding circumstances as well as the addiction itself, it is incredibly important to remember that there is no singular answer or approach. You will see this repeated often throughout these pages, and for good reason. We are all vastly diverse individuals - whether we are talking about siblings, spouses, or strangers. It is precisely because of these differences that there cannot be an unchanging, concrete way to handle the road to recovery for someone struggling with the challenges of addiction. While there will be many different lessons and points made as we continue, every single word is meant to be adapted to your personal situation.

Perhaps there is a section that speaks particularly to you; do not be afraid to spend extra time on those areas. Take extensive notes. Use this book as source material for further research. However you go about it, you should always give yourself the freedom to experience this guideline in a way that you can relate to. In the same way, there might be parts that you do not feel any connection with, nor do you feel it is advantageous to your recovery program. That is also perfectly okay! You are building a new life, so you and your support group will know the best methods and areas which need the most focus.

Personalize everything as you can! *You* are the focus. *You* have the liberty to adjust and adapt where needed, as long as your health and well-being are the priority.

SYMPTOMS OF ADDICTION

There are many indicators that a person is suffering from addiction. It is important to recognize the signs of possible dependence in order to properly work on yourself. A person suffering from some form of substance disorder may develop a sudden lack of self-control, or they may find that they are unable to stop the addictive behavior; these are examples of symptoms. With every decision you make along this journey, you are being given another tool that will be vital in having a full, well-rounded life.

The subsequent paragraphs will discuss some possible symptoms of addiction.

Lack of Control

A major symptom of addiction is a lack of self-control. You may find that you want to reduce your consumption of alcohol, or maybe you want to limit the hours you spend playing video games, but you can't.

Even though you regret it, you just cannot stop yourself from engaging in that activity or consuming that substance. Feeling like you have lost control is a major cause of addiction, as well as the groundwork for other signs of addiction. Awareness of self and being able to cultivate self-control is an essential part of freedom.

It is important to uncover the difference between *willpower* and *self-control*. A commonly accepted concept within the realm of psychology is that willpower leads to - or is a catalyst to - self-control. In 2011, Americans considered the chief reason they didn't achieve their goals to be directly attributed to their willpower[1]. In that same vein of thinking, losing self-control will gradually erode the strength of that will. By viewing it from the perspective of the two being in a balanced, symbiotic relationship, you can be aware enough to sense when something is off with either - or both.

Loss of Interest in Other Activities

Oftentimes, people who struggle with addiction find it difficult to maintain or build up interests. This is usually because, over time, the only activities they would engage in would involve the harmful substance or activities that fuel their addiction. They tend to neglect such activities because they neither encourage the activity nor the use of the substance. If you constantly put off recreational, educational, or social activities because you want to use a substance or engage in an activity that you are dependent on, you are most likely addicted. This loss of interest in non-addiction related activities sometimes destroys the relationships in your life.

In actuality, what occurs is not so much a *loss* of interest, but more a transfer. That time in your life prior to when addiction was in charge, you found joy and that interest in the activity itself, including the actions, the social aspect, or simply being able to relax and separate from stress. Once that dependence crept in, you found those same areas of fulfillment, but *solely* in the addiction. You simply moved where your enthusiasm was, and a part of recovery and learning how to live a new life means finding a way to move it back.

This is also a pertinent subject to bring up concerning the recovery process itself. A loss of interest is a very common red flag as an indication of a deeper issue, but the subject of "interests" will also come into play later. Consider now, as a starter, what activities or hobbies have drawn your interest as you began your recovery, and now wherever you are in your timeline? Life is about more than survival, as you are discovering, and part of that journey is enjoyment.

Negative Effects on Social Life and Relationships

Addiction has negative consequences on your life, this has been a frequently discussed concept already. People who struggle with this disorder may lash out at others, especially at those in their lives who have noticed their dependency on substances and/or activities that are negatively impacting their lives. They may also experience mood swings and massive blows to their self-esteem. This is because they often feel guilt about their addiction but are unable to stop themselves. If you are going through this, you are not alone.

It is the secrecy that tends to increase the negative effects on you and those around you. There is a significant burden that rests on the mind when you have to literally split your life in two: one portion that must effectively hide the usage while still maintaining it, and the other part that has to act normal in social situations. Trying to juggle these partitions of self becomes exhausting, and can also create a sense of paranoia. If *you* know everything that is going on, then every action or word someone says to you could be misconstrued as suspicion or accusation. This puts the addicted person on a constant defensive stance, leading to more exhaustion, and eventually to the lashing out we discussed above.

Significant Energy Spent on Secrecy

Addiction is a truly tiring condition that leaves a person feeling drained. You are constantly hiding your addiction from people because you do not want them to know what you are going through. You may even become paranoid when they start asking questions about your loss of weight, or any other obvious physical signs of your addiction, mostly because it is connected to your use. Addiction and secrecy are dangerous because the continued consumption of the addictive substance or engagement in the habit-forming behavior often has negative consequences. Secrecy while attempting to stop using drugs or alcohol can lead to death.

Increased Tendency to Take Risks

When a person is addicted, they will do almost anything to get their "fix." The possibility of taking risks increases on two fronts: the need to access the activity or substance, and the need to use or engage without being caught. People struggling with addiction push their limits every time they use the substance or engage in the activity they are addicted to. Have you ever come up with an elaborate scheme to avoid getting caught while using?

The next stage of this is what ends up creating the longevity of an addiction, and that is scheming to get away with it. When you manage to avoid consequence the first time you take a risk - stealing, lying, etc. - the reward can be as immediate and fulfilling as the substance itself. You are aware that in order to continue this system of using, the act you just undertook will most likely have to be repeated. Because this is an established fact, realizing that you got away with it will create a false sense of being untouchable, thus that may be the trigger for the increase in risk. Remember that addiction will *never* plateau, which is why it is not a viable treatment and is simply a mask. Every rung you climb on the risk ladder will lead upwards to another more difficult, more damaging one, until you either fall or begin to climb back down.

Withdrawal Symptoms

The most difficult part of addiction is quitting. The thing about addiction is that cessation of the use of the substance or cessation of the activity itself causes emotional and physical trauma. You may have tried to quit feeding your addiction once or twice but you could not get through nausea, anxiety, sweats, and other withdrawal symptoms. It is not easy to overcome addiction by oneself, especially substance addiction.

Just like the patterns that assisted in getting you to this point, once you start to give in it will naturally become easier. This can also create a cycle, one that emerges each time you consider getting clean. It is okay to admit fear when you consider the true depth of withdrawals, but it is also necessary to know the good health and positive promises that come from getting through it. There has to be belief, both in yourself and in the process, for it to be effective and for you to be willing to undertake the challenge.

Tolerance

The more a person consumes substances, or engages in behaviors that are addictive, the greater the amount they need to appease the body's learned appetite. For example, when a person keeps overeating, their brain releases dopamine to reinforce the connection between food and pleasure, thus causing them to eat even more, even more often. When they continue that cycle, their brain continues releasing high amounts of dopamine. The body recognizes an improper balance going on, and tries to repair the irregularity by regulating the amount of dopamine and starts producing less. This becomes an issue because their brain still requires a certain amount of dopamine to function properly. The body makes up for the lesser than normal dopamine by causing them to crave food, knowing from experience that this increased intake can rectify the situation.

In effect, you are putting your mind and body at war with one another, and sometimes within the same factions. Both systems are dedicated to balance, but as these distortions of the status quo continue, they will be forced to adjust. The body is a truly incredible machine, and when a foreign operation is introduced the internal procedures are thrown off kilter.

TYPES OF ADDICTION

Although most people consider substance addiction to refer to a singular idea or singular kind of addiction, there are two recognized types of addiction: Behavioral Addiction and Substance Addiction. Both of these two versions affect individuals differently, as with the other symptoms of the affliction itself. One person may have a tendency to turn to one substance and one substance only, while another ends up developing an addiction to both a behavior and a substance, while a third example could show a person having a completely different experience altogether with addiction. When dealing with something as deeply complex as the subject of addiction, it is important to recognize the fluidity of the impacts. There is a required respect that comes with the territory, and in this instance you must respect the impossibility in having a singular approach to this issue.

Because of this, let's observe the different variations that occur when discussing addiction:

Behavioral Addiction

Behavioral Science experts determined that anything that is capable of causing dependence through stimulation can be an addiction. When behaviors become compulsory and obligatory, they inch toward being under the umbrella definition of an addiction. Behavioral dependency may be harder to notice than substance addiction because it is incredibly common to mistake this variation for an obsessive interest. While you could be considered a "super fan" or over-the-top, when the actions fall under a more social category, they can be seen as simply habits that many people engage in. Most people would not bat an eyelid at someone who is always on the internet, or someone who is always shopping. When someone's hygiene and self-image begin to suffer from a dependence on the internet, or when severe financial disruption occurs due to one's obsession with shopping, those are red flags.

Behavioral addictions such as internet browsing, overeating, shopping, gambling, sex and pornography, overworking, and many more, are too often seen as outside the realm of addiction because the individual is addicted to the particular behavior or the feeling attached to it. Unfortunately, in these cases, the problem isn't seen until it reaches an extreme level. Just like any other disease, addiction can be fatal or have permanent damage if left until the advanced stages.

The National Council on Problem Gambling reported that more than 2 percent of Americans are addicted to gambling. The 5th edition of the Diagnostic and Statistical Manual of Mental Disorders (DSM-V) recognizes gambling addiction as the only non-substance addiction. There are still disagreements as to whether behaviors and habits can be causes of addiction. This is because there are still debates about which activities can become addictive, and there is yet to be an agreed-upon point at which behaviors become addictions. Although, as stated above, the stance commonly taken by professionals is that if a behavior *can* be classified as causing dependence, it can also be seen as an addictive action.

The lack of peer-reviewed scientific evidence is the reason for its exclusion from the DSM-V. Regardless of the lack of scientific diagnosis, many people struggle with behavioral addictions. People struggling with behavioral addiction often find that their relationships with people are negatively affected. More often than not, they may have serious financial repercussions and problems.

While it is known that there is a vilified stigma around the term *addiction*, it is important to also recognize when real, presenting issues of dependence arise in the behavioral form that they are often shrugged off. There seems to be a subconscious need to rate the types of addiction, and therefore rank where you prioritize them. Drugs and other substances are more mainstream in their coverage, so when they are present in the real world the reaction is more sympathetic. On the other hand, when the presentation is on the side of behavior, the reaction is much less understanding. In fact, I have heard reasonings to dismiss these cases due to the fact that they would distract from "actual addiction problems."

Dealing with addiction demands compassion, and part of that is the removal of these dangerous and destructive stereotypes and assumptions. There is a good chance that an addict has not felt much acceptance during their struggles, and by viewing their real pain and challenges in an unsympathetic manner will do untold damage to an already lost person.

Substance Addiction

This is the commonly accepted type of addiction. Substance addiction is the dependence on any chemical intoxicant or substance. Addiction to substances such as alcohol, cocaine, cannabis, and opioids have a very high chance of causing dependency. The Diagnostic and Statistical Manual of Mental Disorders (DSM-V) recommends the term substance use disorder when dealing with substance addiction.

The DSM-V classifies drugs into ten separate classes and recognizes substance use disorders that could arise from the use of these drugs. The ten classes of drugs are thus: alcohol; tobacco; cannabis; inhalants; opioids; hallucinogens (such as LSD, phencyclidine, and others); stimulants (such as cocaine, and amphetamine-type substances); hypnotics, sedatives, and anxiolytics; caffeine; and unknown substances. It is important to not simply pass over that information because, as we discussed earlier, the subject of addiction - any type of addiction - requires both seeing the depth of information at hand and the importance of understanding the different variations rather than generalizing.

Substance addiction often has physical and psychological impacts upon the individual. In regards to the physical consequences, constant consumption of alcohol could cause inflammation of the liver, damage to the pancreas, permanent brain dysfunction, and lengthy list of other physical harms. Addiction to alcohol could also put a person at a higher risk of pneumonia, along with the damaging of the heart and liver. Pregnant women who remain addicted to alcohol put their unborn child at risk of having Fetal Alcohol Syndrome. Fetal alcohol syndrome (FAS) is a condition that occurs in children who were exposed to alcohol while in the womb. It causes growth problems and brain damage.

In 2017, over 180,000 people died from alcohol disorder, making it the highest cause of death among other substance use disorders. Despite this fact, and that the statistics have been available for some time, it remains incredibly difficult to maintain distance from alcohol in today's world. Not only that, but the reaction in social situations to someone who no longer partakes is rarely positive, and usually uncomfortable. The widespread availability of alcohol creates a dangerous environment to the members of society who suffer from the affliction.

The psychological consequences of substance addiction revolve around mental health. Many people who are addicted to substances are diagnosed with mental disorders. Substance addiction causes changes in the brain, and these changes could lead to depression, hallucinations, anxiety, and other problems. In the same line of thought, when dealing with those who have a long-term addiction, the withdrawals alone could lead to these disorders. While the full impact of this type of continued abuse remains unknown, what we do know shows a need for as much healing as possible, while realizing the serious nature of the circumstance.

Similarities Between the Types of Addiction

Generally, behavioral and substance addiction share similar reactions from the brain. In both types of addiction, continued use or engagement causes the brain to require more in order to avoid withdrawal symptoms. Tolerance is a shared result of both types of addiction. Another similarity is the general lack of interest in activities other than those which encourage their addiction. For example, someone who is addicted to cocaine will most likely lose interest in anything that is not cocaine. The same goes for someone who is addicted to watching television; they will most likely be hooked to their TVs, rather than anything else.

People who are addicted to substances or activities tend to lose self-control. This lack of self-control is a major driving force for the two types of addiction. This loss of self-control is evident in the need to continue using, despite the negative consequences of addiction in a person's life.

Differences Between the Types of Addiction

The major difference between substance addiction and behavioral addiction is that, in the former, the individual is addicted to a substance while the latter sees the individual addicted to a particular behavior or the feeling that comes with indulging in such behavior.

The physical signs of substance addiction are often absent in cases of behavioral addiction. For instance, some physical signs that indicate the use of cannabis and other cannabis-containing substances are red eyes and dry mouth. These physical signs would not be present in a person struggling with exercise addiction.

Another variation is the approach that is usually taken in regards to these two, as we briefly touched on earlier. Since substance addiction is the more visible or recognizable of the two, it is given more validity compared to a behavioral type of addiction. While it is important to understand the issue of addiction as a whole, it cannot be done without also seeing the individual impacts and characteristics associated with each specific case. Above all, never get to a point where you only see an issue or a disease, especially with yourself! The people behind those labels and variations are the focus, *you* are the focus. Well being, health, and stability, those are the goals, no matter what kind of an addiction you are dealing with.

THE BIOLOGY OF ADDICTION: HOW DOES IT WORK?

If you are struggling with addiction, you may have tried to quit, and if it did not take then it would have been difficult for you. You may have lost your friends or family, maybe even your job or a scholarship. You are not happy about the way you are but you don't know how to stop. Why is it so difficult to quit? Why do you keep going back, even though you know better?

We've discussed some of the mental aspects of addiction, but when it comes to biology, it is a compilation of a few different systems. Your mind understands at least some of the danger you continue to put yourself in, but that occurs while your body is demanding that you satiate the craving. When that isn't fulfilled, you experience both physical and emotional trauma from the sudden deficiency of the substance in your body. When this cycle is repeated enough, using the addiction as treatment, the mind begins to alter its stance and the voices of reason become dimmer. After a while you will have your body and mind working together in a continuous structure designed around addiction fulfillment.

The use of medicine for the treatment of addiction seems counterintuitive to some but scientists have shown that treatments can control the need for substances. Having a dependency is a long-lasting condition affecting both mind and body, and that is why people who successfully quit are never fully free from the danger of returning to addiction. The biology of this process proves that people need more than just willpower and determination to overcome these challenges and afflictions. The more addicted or dependent a person is to a substance or an activity, the more changes happen within the brain. It takes a lot of work and time for the brain to return to its normal state and, unfortunately, in some cases there really is no going back.

Your body is incredibly adept at healing: from bones to muscle and even types of nerves will regrow, sometimes stronger than before. The brain, however, is a much more fragile system. The toll your body undergoes during the addiction usually reveals itself in time, and when you begin to repair yourself, the healing will show in your appearance as well. Your mind is much harder to fix, if it can be fixed at all. This is why there is a sense of urgency when it comes to entering recovery, because each day spent in the cycle of damage could be the day something unfixable ends up being harmed.

The power of addiction is in its ability to control and oftentimes destroy the key areas of the brain involved with our survival. The constant use of drugs can damage the prefrontal cortex, the part of the brain that controls decision-making. As a result of this, people are unable to make the decision to stop using drugs even though they know they consume too much, even though their act of using is damaging their relationships with people, and despite the fact that they realize that they will eventually have to steal to buy drugs, if that isn't already the case.

This damage to the regions of your brain can also cause you to live in multiple worlds. What this means is that you have to justify your actions to yourself somehow, and the further into the addiction you go, the more you need to condone. Because you cannot fully admit the extent of your situation - because then you would have to address it - you need to go to more and more extremes to warrant the actions you take. From this comes an imaginary world of "one day" where all your good choices reside.

One day you'll come clean to everyone, but not now.

One day you will find a way to work through all these issues, but today you just can't.

A healthy brain rewards healthy activities and behaviors such as moderate exercising, swimming, reading, or bonding with people. When a person engages in such productive and robust activities, the brain motivates them to repeat the activities; the brain is incentivizing, really. A healthy mind functions properly, even in times of emergency or danger. Having this positive, strong, active perspective on life prompts immediate reaction to dangerous situations in order to protect you.

In situations that may have negative consequences, the prefrontal cortex decides on the course of action. But when the brain is affected by addiction, especially to an addictive substance, its normal processes can be affected. Addiction can make the danger-sensing parts of the brain go haywire; thus, causing anxiety, stress, and nervousness even when the individual is not using. Addiction can also control the part of the brain responsible for rewarding behaviors, and cause an individual to want more. When people are addicted to substances or behaviors, they often turn to using them to stop from feeling bad, rather than for pleasure.

In fact, over time, the user can experience a "new normal" where life has switched, in a sense. They have used so much that their time spent under the influence now feels normal, while the time in sobriety is uncomfortable and surreal, considering it is usually spent on the search for another fix. While this is not always the case, getting to this point can have lasting effects on how someone views the world.

Scientists have been unable to pinpoint exactly why some people get addicted while others do not. According to the National Institutes of Health, the risk of addiction has a tendency to increase in people whose parents are alcoholics or drug addicts. Addiction is sometimes caused by multiple genes. While scientists have been unable to determine the precise genetic cause, research has shown that genes may have an influence regarding substance use. In fact, scientists have estimated the influence of genetics in causing addiction occurs in nearly 60 percent of studied cases. It is important to note that the risk of addiction from certain genes does not mean that every member of a family will be affected. This is a fluctuating science that has very little concrete information at this time, and as such should be handled with both care and patience.

Our genes, however, are not the only factor that increases the risk of possible addiction. People who grew up around addicts are also at a higher chance of becoming addicts themselves. Also, children who come from homes that normalize physical and mental abuse are at higher risk of becoming addicted to substances. The earlier a person starts consuming substances such as alcohol and cocaine, the greater the likelihood of addiction.

In essence, when someone spends their formative years in an environment of fear or trauma, the desire to escape this reality will be present from an early stage. While the reasons for the turn to addiction differs from person to person, the core desire is to remove oneself from the issues around them, to escape. Consistent immersion in such a negative space from a young age can certainly bring about these circumstances of addiction more expediently, and at a more intense level.

THE EVOLUTION OF ADDICTION

Addiction can be viewed from an evolutionary perspective, as well, in order to discover the causes of substance abuse. This approach to dependency also supports psychological treatment alongside medication, as it aims to prevent substance use disorders. There is significant research that points to the co-evolution of mammalian brains and psychotropic plants, plants that affect a person's mind. Thus, human brains and these specific types of plants affected one another during the process of evolving; these plants were not as potent as they are now, and the human brain developed receptors for the plants.

Evidence for this coevolution is the body's development of defenses against over-toxicity, such as vomiting reflexes.

The early form of humans would collect plants and, as time passed, they learned that some of these plants caused euphoric reactions or contained healing properties. For the plants that had a more intoxicating effect, people would harvest those more than others. Extensive research has shown that in order to cope on an evolutionary scale, there developed an arms race, of sorts. The plant would evolve stronger chemical compounds to dissuade humans from consuming them, and the people would develop a tolerance or learn how to regulate the impact[2]. Some possible examples of this, according to several botanical experts, are nicotine, morphine, and atropine, to name just a few[3].

The human brain is vulnerable to addiction because the parts of the brain that regulate behavior are based on chemical transmitters. It is therefore unsurprising that people get addicted to substances which can easily stimulate the system. The susceptibility of the human brain to addiction is proof that you are not weak because of your addiction, and there are other factors that increase the risk of addiction. When people begin to look at the entire study of dependency from an evolutionary standpoint, they are closer to understanding how to remedy and prevent addiction without only treating the symptoms.

Whether it is evolutionary, genetic, or from a different origin altogether, it is important to think of addiction from every possible perspective. The more you understand the underlying causations, the damage done and subsequent healing, the more this information enables you to be constructive. Recovery is a process, whether it is for you or a loved one. There is a person behind the judgement and vilified stigmas, a person who has seen the lowest places that humanity can go, a person who both deserves and needs love as well as the respect needed to take the time to understand their perspective.

Addiction is a brain condition which has a greater effect worldwide on more people than we are willing to admit. It comes in many forms and, until people address it, it is only going to evolve into more of a problem. In the next chapter, you will learn about how addiction comes to be. How did you become dependent on your addiction? There are many different paths that could have brought you here, and each one comes with its own baggage and differences.

GENERAL POINTS FOR REVIEW

- Addiction has been a problem for multiple eras and generations.
- These are the general signs of addiction: tolerance, lack of control, little to no interest in non-addiction related activities, affected social life, investment of energy on addiction, and withdrawal symptoms.
- Behavioral addiction and substance addiction are the two types of addiction.
- Behavioral addiction is the dependence on particular activities or behaviors.
- Substance addiction is a common type of addiction. It is the dependence on substances such as alcohol, and drugs.
- Addiction affects the brain, and in most cases, medication is the best treatment.

2

HOW ADDICTION HAPPENS

In the first few sections, you were given an in-depth discussion on addiction but you may be curious about how addiction manifests in your life or in the life of someone you know. How does it happen? How did you become this person who functions in such a way that you cannot live without using? People are not born with addictions, nor is someone with an addiction inherently a "bad person." The only situation in which babies are born with prior connection with drugs is when the mother used drugs while pregnant, and even in those circumstances it is not the fault of the child. The point is that there is a point where something indeed changes, and we will explore the different possible ways that alteration came about.

Addiction is not a two-step process, as we talked about before: you do not wake up, drink alcohol, and the next day, you are an alcoholic. Addiction happens over time, and usually only after consistent use of a substance or engagement in an activity. The path to addiction is slippery. One has to learn to draw the line between indulgence and overindulgence to avoid addiction. It is easy for things to get out of hand when you play video games for an hour a day, the next day you might want to play for two hours. The gradual increase could go on from there, and you could become addicted. Even this seems incredibly two dimensional, so we'll try another approach, one with a more personal viewpoint.

I smoked for years, decades actually. The first time I had a cigarette it made me light-headed and I felt nauseous, but my friends had been regular smokers for a few years and I didn't want to look completely foolish in front of them. Because of my incredibly low tolerance, and that I had come from a rather strict upbringing, I was firm about not becoming a "smoker." In my mind, there were several absolutes that separated a "smoker" from someone who casually and occasionally had a cigarette. One big red flag to me was buying a pack, sometimes a carton, and in my eyes that would end it all. Another was owning lighters and having an ashtray. It made sense in my mind that as long I knew the identifiers and maintained a distance from those identifiers, I could have my cake and eat it, too.

At that time, I was struggling with extreme stress and depression, my first real bout with these issues. I didn't drink and drugs were simply something to firmly say *NO* to, as I had learned throughout school. Cigarettes, however, fell somewhere in a gray area as far as I saw it. I was honestly looking for something to provide me with a distraction, not really an "escape" per say, but rather something to release that stress that seemed to have taken up residence in my chest. I didn't buy them so I would only smoke around my friends because I would ask my buddies for a cigarette when I wanted one - which still wasn't very often. My personal situation did not improve, though, and from that came more anxiety and more depression.

The change was so gradual that I didn't even notice it was happening, until one day I realized that I had a drawer with at least four lighters in it, plus two ashtrays. My justifications had been that even if I bent the rules on the outskirts of the risk factor - lighters and ashtrays - I could still avoid ruin by staying away from that core pitfall: buying a pack. You can tell where I am going with this, and within a few weeks I had my first purchased pack, heart crushed, but stress temporarily managed. I was a heavy smoker until very recently, and I still can't recall exactly how I went from getting light-headed to smoking several packs a day. Addiction is not quick, nor is it easy to track. This is something to keep in mind as you continue.

Many people go through rough times and some come out of the experience with scars - mental and physical - from trauma. Society, however, does not encourage people to address their trauma in order to move on with life. Boys and men, as a generalized gender in this case, are told to get over it; they are told to "act like men" so they bottle things up. Women and girls are dismissed as overly emotional. Neither of these cases is true, and both stereotypes are incredibly harmful to the healing process. The expectations on both genders to conduct themselves in a certain, preset manner despite outside events is ridiculous, and will have a lasting impact on a person. Male or female, the devastation caused by addiction is still a real, unbiased consequence.

Ignoring trauma does not make it go away. Instead, it makes the victim deal with the trauma in the worst way. While many victims of trauma end up hurting themselves or others through self-hate or violence, some turn to substance abuse or overindulge in habits and behaviors. While it is true that many aspects of our modern world are learning new, more efficient ways to treat addiction, there are still so many who are overlooked. Silence is never the answer, whether it is about getting yourself the help you need, or it is providing support to a loved one through their struggles. No one will make it through alone.

Many people use these substances and habits as coping mechanisms. They rarely have a plan in place to deal with their trauma. Instead, they usually aim to run away from it. Addiction, for many people, is a way to hide from pain and trauma; addiction is a tool for escape. It is easy to turn away from your problems, and even easier to depend on behaviors or substance use. The issue of dependency is a form of self-medication for many. It stems from the human tendency to run away from problems, rather than addressing and overcoming them. This is one of the reasons that addiction continues to thrive in society. If we were better at recognizing and then healing or dealing with our problems in healthier ways, maybe addiction would not be such a prominent issue in our society.

Addiction starts when your brain convinces you that you can not live without depending on a substance or habit. When you start taking a substance or engaging in activities that are potentially addictive, your brain encourages you to continue doing those things. As explained in the previous chapter, your brain releases dopamine when you engage in activities that it finds pleasurable. The brain releases this chemical when you hang out with friends, or read novels, or generally do things that are healthy and enjoyable to you, personally. Your brain does this to encourage you to do those things again; an incentive to live in a way that is conducive to overall health. However, when you continually use, your brain produces excess dopamine. This, in turn, causes your brain to reduce the production of dopamine - even though your body needs a certain level of dopamine to properly function. Your body makes up for the lack of dopamine by causing you to consistently use. At this point, a chemical switch occurs in our brain and we begin to depend on our addiction, believing that we need it to function.

Addiction is harmful to us physically and mentally but it can also affect those we love. Addiction drives people to do things they normally would not have done if they were not addicted. Oftentimes, people who are addicted sacrifice their love for themselves and others in pursuit of their vice. You may find that you lie to your partner about how you spend your money, or you may push your parents out of your life because they seem suspicious of your activities. Or maybe you borrowed some money from a friend to buy alcohol, and you know you hardly ever borrow money. It is through these seemingly little things that addiction begins to lead you astray.

This is why it is so important to maintain a stance of awareness when it comes to the subject of addiction and dependency. You know how you usually act, and you know what drives those actions. When something occurs that causes you to act outside of those usual parameters, it should be recognized and addressed. What happens instead is you ignore it the first time, or even the first few times it arises. You figure it was a rough day, or just an anomaly. It was nothing to take seriously, because when you stop and actually look the situation over, you are well aware of what you will find. By remaining in that place of awareness, you are able to notice when these out-of-personality changes occur, and recognize your patterns in order to stop the negative cycles or spirals before they take hold.

How does addiction begin to take over our lives? This hostile and destructive process usually starts from our biological side before it advances to our emotional side. Many people assume that addicts are people who lack self-control or are selfish, but research conducted in the last sixty years has proven that addiction has more to do with a person's biology than their will. It is easier to understand addiction when we realize that our human biology causes us to seek out things that are pleasurable to us. We can rise above our biology, however; this is where psychological, and societal factors come in. We are not slaves to our biology and that is why people can recover from addiction. This makes dependency similar to other diseases such as diabetes in that living a healthy lifestyle can help manage such afflictions. Research has shown that, like other diseases, some people are genetically predisposed to addiction.

While it is well known that the increase of dopamine upon constant use is what causes the "buzz" or reward that we chase after, recent research has shown another critical role dopamine plays in addiction. There are specific dopamine receptors that are responsible for the motivation to forgo instant gratification in order to work toward a greater reward. These dopamine receptors are also called D2 receptors and they are located in a region of the brain called the striatum. A lower dopamine response among D2 receptors can cause people to chase short-term rewards, and instant gratification – both of which are common behaviors in people with addiction disorders. Some people have fewer D2 receptors in their striatum, making them genetically predisposed to addiction. Those people with lower D2 receptors are more prone to impulsivity. On the other hand, there are people with higher D2 receptors who tend to be more successful in treating addiction from the perspective of behavior, i.e. through behavioral interventions. Some people have reduced D2 receptors not because they were born that way but as a result of constant use of substances or engagement in certain behaviors and activities that prompt a higher-than-normal release of dopamine. When the brain inevitably regulates the dopamine levels, the level of D2 receptors available in the striatum reduces, and those with addiction become even more likely to use and more impulsive.

The human brain, our mind, is a very complex organ. When our brains function properly, we are able to adapt to our environment with healthy coping mechanisms. It is this very adaptability of the brain that can have the potential to contribute to addiction. Having this affliction changes the brain's structures and its functions, as well as your ability to maintain a natural balance. Addiction also alters the brain's chemistry, causing damage that, in some cases, can be irreversible. Many of the symptoms associated with addiction are present as a result of these changes in the way your synapses are firing. For example, the brain's cerebral cortex is in charge of regulating potentially damaging behaviors such as compulsivity, impulsivity, and decision-making. When you constantly engage in pleasure-inducing activities such as drug use, gambling, or shopping, your cerebral cortex changes. This makes it less capable of preventing negative impulses, and you will have more difficulty resisting the urge to use.

The hypothalamus is a part of the brain that includes autonomic regulatory centers that regulate reactions such as stress. Substance use affects the hypothalamus' ability to regulate these reactions, causing people to use even more in order to relieve reactions such as stress, and fight-or-flight. When someone tries to withdraw from substance use, they are flooded with stress thus creating a vicious cycle. Another symptom of addiction that is caused by changes in the brain is the memories and cues associated with activities and the withdrawal symptoms that are triggered by discontinuing use. The brain's amygdala is associated with memories, cues, and emotion. The brain associates certain memories with certain cues, and any attempt to dissociate from such cues causes withdrawal. For example, if someone drinks alcohol every time they get home from work, the brain associates coming home from work as a cue to drink alcohol. This cue is stored alongside the positive memory associated with drinking alcohol. An attempt to stop drinking alcohol can cause withdrawal. The memory of withdrawal is unpleasant enough to serve as a powerful cue to continue the addictive behavior.

EMOTIONAL CONSEQUENCES OF ADDICTION

Addiction, over time, causes emotional instability in the life of someone struggling with addiction, and by extension causes instability in the lives of their loved ones. This type of mental disruption is dangerous because it can worsen a person's addiction and cause their lives to be taken over by their need to fulfill their dependent mind and body. It may not seem like it but people struggling with addiction often feel similar emotions with their loved ones. Loved ones of addicts often struggle with guilt and the feeling that they could have done more to prevent the addiction. Addicts often feel guilty about their addiction disorder, despite their inability to stop using.

The range of emotions linked with the entire process could stretch endlessly. It is because of the incredible complexity of the circumstances that the reactions of everyone involved run so high, both the reactions of the addict and the reactions of those who are trying to support them. It is not a low stakes situation, and will bring out depths of people that may not have been present previously. When something or someone people love is threatened, they will go to many extremes to ensure the safety of that subject. In this case it is how much those involved - including yourself - are going to let themselves be emotionally present.

Guilt

People who are addicted usually feel guilty for their behavior. For some people, they may experience guilt while using while others may experience guilt after using. During sober periods, or when they are done with the activity, they may experience guilt for the questionable behaviors they engaged in while using. They may feel guilty for making their loved ones suffer, whether physically, financially, or emotionally. Guilt is a dangerous emotion because the loved ones may attempt to make up for their guilt by enabling the addict. This will only worsen and complicate things.

This is one of the more driving forces behind many different aspects of the process. Guilt is a powerful emotion, a powerful force in general, and can either be a brilliantly positive catalyst or have an incredibly detrimental impact. The person who is dealing with an addiction most likely feels extensive guilt over what they are doing, but this does not always mean they will suddenly come to terms with what needs to be done. In fact, more often than not, people use this onset of guilt to shrink further into themselves, usually resulting in returning to the addiction - sometimes harder than before. This is why an approach that has guilt as a focus is rarely the right step to take. This "tough love" method can be useful in certain situations, but when improperly implemented, it can severely damage already harmed relationships and further affirm to the addict that their dependency is the only constant.

Helplessness

An addict may feel helpless because they do not know how to quit using. They may feel overwhelmed because they want to stop without help from anyone, but they cannot. Many addicts feel powerless and it is not uncommon for them to simply accept their situation. At the same time, the family and friends of an addict may feel like they are also helpless and unable to solve their loved one's afflictions to being dependent. Even though this group of people know that they did not cause the addiction, they know that they cannot control it either, and that does not make them feel any less helpless.

As with guilt, this can be a very powerful factor. There are few emotions as empty as *helplessness* feels. It can bring on a plethora of over-emotional forces - the aforementioned guilt, anger, self-loathing, to name a few - and the end result would be incredibly overwhelming. In truth, the only way to combat feeling helpless is to discover what *will* help. Usually the reason the loved ones feel this way is because they want to be the ones fixing the situation, the ones being there for the addicted party. Because they must rely on an outside source, or simply one that isn't them, they feel like they didn't assist whatsoever.

On the other side is the person struggling with their addiction. The feeling of helplessness is a constant already, and seeing the effect it has on their loved ones only increases that. Because of the destructive cycle they are in, their response to this situation is skewed. Rather than being able to think through the possible solutions, the mere idea of coming to terms with their issue brings on more isolation. From that comes more of the same cycle, thus producing more helpless moments.

Shame[1]

Shame is commonly felt by people struggling with addiction, as well as by their loved ones. This deep-rooted emotion can make a person feel less worthy than they actually are. It convinces us that we have less value than we do because of the situation we find ourselves in. This is how shame can eat away at an addict and those in their different circles. Because many people equate addiction with moral weakness or lack of self-control, people struggling with addiction, and those around them, can feel embarrassed to speak out.

Often the terms *shame* and *guilt* are used interchangeably, but they should be looked at and utilized separately. While both are very real and exist throughout the environments of addiction, they represent two very different emotions that originate from separate sources.

Guilt arises from feeling remorse, usually regarding an action you participated in or caused. This is a more internalized emotion, focused on what was done wrong and how *you* feel about it. The presence of guilt is not always a negative thing, and can actually be proof that you have sensitivity to the feelings of others.

Shame, however, is a much more painful, visceral feeling. Whereas guilt was about *what* you had done, the shame is due to the pain you caused *from* that action. It is an awareness that you conducted yourself improperly, and thus are going through a form of self punishment to mentally rectify the situation.

Both of these emotions regularly exist during the difficult process associated with addiction, but it is important to know the difference between the two and how they relate to ourselves, and the situation as a whole.

Sadness

Sadness is a very prevalent emotion in the life of an addict. People struggling with addiction may be sad about the opportunities they have missed out on because of their addiction. Or they may be sad about expectations they failed to meet. Their loved ones may be feeling this way because they witness how addiction limits the life of the person they care about. However it occurs, this should be an expected occurrence at some point - or many - throughout this process.

Feeling sad over something is a more reactionary emotion than an origin. For example, guilt and shame, respectively, may *bring on* feeling sad. You first must realize and understand that a situation is not what it could be, or that something is lacking, and then the sadness comes.

Fear

Fear is a very real part of the life of an addict and their loved ones. No matter how inconsequential or complex these fears are, they can negatively impact the decisions and thoughts of addicts and their loved ones. The extreme worries of addicts may revolve around their use – specifically where and when they can get their next fix. The similar feelings of the loved ones of addicts can range from fear of financial problems to broken relationships to incarceration or death.

A very dangerous situation can arise as time passes in regards to this fear. Each time you choose your addiction over a more positive option, you slowly wear down the voices of goodness and health that are trying to tell you otherwise. These, along with the other influences in your mind, are necessary to creating a positive method of living. Without fear, especially, you create a lifestyle where there is no consequence, no deterrent to the negative actions that are being done. Courage and bravery do not exist without fear, just as the ability to know where danger lies is also from having a healthy sense of fear.

It is very difficult to break free of addiction. For some people, once the negative spiral into addiction has been initiated, it becomes very difficult to get out of it. For many of the afflicted who struggle with substance abuse, it is very easy to lose that grip on reality. Constant use of alcohol or drugs can shorten the time an addict spends sober and free of the influence of their use. While it is more difficult for people who are addicted to behaviors to lose track of reality, it is not impossible. When a person spends hours on end cooped up in their room playing video games, they often lose track of reality. They may not know what time it is or even remember what they were going to do before they started playing. The same can apply to gamble addicts. They may gamble and lose track of time, or how much money they have spent.

Another way to look at it is that, for most people who struggle with addiction, there is nothing on the other side. While those who are trying to help them continue to reference how amazing it will be once sobriety is reached, and share success stories about a new, fresh life, this engagement is usually met with skepticism from the addicted party. Even the concept of a life free from the dependency is a distant dream, if it is still one at all. When those loved ones in the innermost circle speak of that "other side," the message falls on deaf ears. The miscommunication occurs because the addict does not want to stir up trouble, or endure the testimonials for much longer, so they respond in a positive, welcoming manner. This causes the supporting group to feel heard, and leave it alone for the time being, allowing the afflicted person more time away from the situation and finding solace in that escapism thought process.

It has to be real to them, the reward factor, and the promise. An addict makes ten thousand broken promises to themselves on a daily basis, so the idea of *something better* just over the horizon is a placation used to justify, rather than a reality of any sort. That is where the true challenge lies: how do you get that person to believe that there is something good, something better, waiting for them in sobriety. The unfortunate truth is that more often than not it takes the exact opposite. Rather than believing that something better was there, a painful rock bottom is reached, and from that comes the crossroads of a lifetime.

Oftentimes, addiction progresses from mere use or activity to the rationale for an action. When you start using cocaine because you do not think you can survive without it, or you need it to get through your day, you are truly addicted. The "birth" of addiction is when your logic is abandoned and your reason for an action is skewed in favor of your use. Addiction does not occur instantaneously; it is an accumulation of things that we have done over time. We often ignore these things or think them too innocuous so we charge ahead without healing from or reflecting on them. These things can be daily consumption of alcohol, or regular shopping, or even overly constant consumption of pornography and other sex-related content.

Everything in this process comes down to one key factor: awareness. Without awareness, you cannot hope to recognize the red flags or the opportunities for change. Without awareness you will not be able to see outside the haze of addiction. Without being aware, you cannot trust in those you love. Learn to trust beyond your perspective, and see through their eyes. It all starts with the ability to be mindful and aware. From that point forward there will certainly be challenges, but you will be prepared to face them with courage and resilience.

GENERAL POINTS FOR REVIEW

- Escapism and the refusal to address our problems can lead to addiction.
- Addiction begins to lead us astray when we dismiss our inhibitions to use, and we start feeling like we cannot survive without using.
- Addiction is not always a lack of self-control or will.
- Some people are genetically predisposed to addiction.
- Addiction causes changes to the brain's chemistry and these changes are the reason for many symptoms associated with addiction.
- Addiction emotionally affects addicts and their loved ones.
- Some emotions that are common between those struggling with addiction and their loved ones are fear, guilt, shame, etc.

3

UNDERSTANDING THE PAST IN ORDER TO BUILD A FUTURE

Addiction is a byproduct of unaddressed trauma and emotional pain. It manifests as a result of unaddressed and unresolved issues of the past. If you have financial issues that threaten to overwhelm you, you may choose to drink your way out of your problems rather than facing them head-on. Your financial issues are not going to disappear out of the blue. What happens is that you abandon addressing those issues for alcohol consumption which can lead to addiction. You need to understand and dissect your problems if you want to overcome addiction. The past is not to be run from, neither is it to be ignored and treated like it does not exist. But you should never dwell in the past. Dwelling in the past will most likely stunt your growth and progress. Far too many people get stuck fighting their past that they forget, or are incapable of, building their future.

Have you, since you decided to either begin the road to recovery, or to help a loved one on their path, examined the full origin of this particular addiction? I am sure that to one extent or another you have examined the factors that led to the various stages of your life, both in and out of the addiction cycle. Have you *truly*, from an almost academic viewpoint, stepped back and looked at the scope of your timeline?

Few people have, and that is because it requires increasing levels of honesty with yourself. You cannot have understanding, especially of your past, without the ability to be vulnerable and transparent. There are most likely some very serious issues that will present themselves through the events you have gone through, and without the permission to be that direct with yourself, it may end up just being a date and a label.

Your past is what it is. While that may seem simplistic, that is a good place to start. You can't alter your past, and even if you suddenly had no cravings, no hardships from the fallout, or any consequence to your life of addiction, you still wouldn't have erased or rewritten what has already been done. Too often this is misconstrued when people take on the path of recovery. They expect that somehow this new life of sobriety comes with a massive, time travelling eraser. You don't get that kind of a re-do, but you do get the chance to ensure the mistakes you made are turned into productive and positive results. *That* is the truth to hold onto. Set out to change your future, but do it from a position of learning from the past - not fighting it.

In order to overcome addiction, you need to find a balance between your past and your future. You need to properly, deeply, understand your past if you want to heal. If you simply forget about your past, you will not be able to rectify anything properly. The further you get into this process, you will find that your hindsight is not nearly as bleak. Whereas before you may have only looked back with shame or disgust, now you see the events that took place all had a part to play in forming who you are now. While you are probably not proud of those moments, you can find peace in knowing you are now taking those errors and relearning habits.

What does it mean to heal? Healing is overcoming and restoring oneself to wellness. True and honest healing purges you of the turmoil you went through in the past. It does not erase where you came from, but it makes things easy to bear. Finding a remedy is a byproduct of addressing the emotions and turmoil that you have been avoiding. It is important to know that with healing comes acceptance of oneself, of what is and has been.

The most powerful thing you can do on your journey to a life free of addiction is to resolve your past. Finding resolution to your past is to successfully accept that you do indeed have one, and understand that you deserve to move forward from it. The first step to take in resolving your past is acceptance.

ACCEPTANCE

Acceptance of oneself is key to true healing. What it means in this sense does not only refer to acknowledging your addiction and deciding that you cannot change; it means recognizing that you have issues and are addicted but you love yourself. In acceptance, loving yourself means you are going to do the best you can to become the best you can be. This begins with seeing the problems, and then formulating a plan knowing that you are going to overcome addiction.

Acceptance will change the way you see yourself and rid you of what is known as a "victim mentality." Victim mentality is a personality trait in which a person blames other people for the problems and challenges they face. People with this type of negative mentality do not own up to their faults, and they deflect responsibility for their actions from themselves to others. Oftentimes, people with victim mentality gain pleasure from being persecuted or pitied. Many people who struggle with addiction have a victim mentality. If you are such a person, you need to take responsibility for your addiction and cast off your victim mentality. When you do this, it becomes easier to free yourself of blame, as you free others of blame. All the resentment you feel toward yourself will drain away upon acceptance of who you are, and what you are going through.

This is a very difficult cycle to break as well, and you should not feel dismissive when it comes to the actual work involved. In order to maintain a life of addiction and dependency, there is at least a modicum of a victim's mentality required to justify the constant battle of self that goes on. While it is factual and known somewhere in your mind that you are not the victim in this scenario, you *have to* convince yourself of that in order to function. You cannot live in a state of refusal to give up your vice, maintain that you are the victim, and still claim stability without having that altered and skewed perspective. It is also for these very reasons that it is absolutely vital to not only fully recognize that pattern, but to reverse that thinking to properly see where either blame or responsibility truly lie.

FORGIVENESS

Forgiveness is the intentional process of letting go of one's feelings of anger, resentment, bitterness, and the need for vengeance toward someone who has hurt us, including ourselves. To be honest, especially in these situations, forgiveness most definitely includes ourselves. In some cases, forgiveness is more for you than it is for another person. Even in situations where someone offends or hurts you, forgiveness is a way for you to move on from that situation. Forgiving yourself allows you to let go of whatever guilt is weighing you down and delaying your journey to an addiction-free life. By forgiving yourself, you find gratitude and happiness even in the darkest of past times.

The ability to forgive is a character strength that more people should strive for. Some people are naturally more forgiving than others because of their personality but this should not deter you from improving your ability to forgive, especially if this is a trait that is difficult for you. People find it difficult to release themselves from that burden because they believe they do not deserve happiness. Other people may find it easy to forgive those who hurt them but are unable to forgive themselves for their past. It is because of all these factors that they may be unable to forgive themselves for their addiction because, as addicts, they believe they will relapse.

The key to moving on from addiction is to remember to always forgive yourself. Remember that your past happened and you cannot change it; what you can change is your future. You must choose to always forgive yourself for your past decisions if you want to move on to a healthier lifestyle. Forgiving yourself does not mean that you condone your past decisions, neither does it mean that you are excusing your actions in the past. It simply means that you have acknowledged your addiction, and you are ready to let go of the negative feelings and thoughts that you have toward yourself as a result of your past addiction. To properly forgive yourself, you have to accept your addiction. When this subject was studied, the results showed that forgiveness may sometimes involve grieving for what was lost. You may have lost your job, your family, or your finances. It is okay to accept what you lost because of your addiction and forgive yourself.

In my experience, when dealing with those who struggle with addiction, they are so hesitant to forgive themselves because they feel that not doing so is a form of penance. This is their way of making up for the time they wasted, the hurt they caused; in effect, it is a trade. They made a ruin of the time they were given, so now that they have found a life of sobriety - despite that, actually - they now must sacrifice peace to atone for the sins of their past. This is not only a severely incorrect way to view the situation, but it is also incredibly damaging. The entire point of emerging whole and new, after the harrowing experiences that brought you here, is to rediscover the inherent value that you possess. Among a list of other things, you gave up that value to yourself when you made damaging decisions after damaging decisions. The truth that you refuse to allow in is that it was *only to you* that your value had diminished. Public opinion be damned, because your worth never faltered and it is a heartbreaking situation indeed when the collateral damage to the choices you made ends up being the existence of any self-worth, esteem and pride.

Forgiveness is very beneficial to you and those you love. By forgiving yourself, you give yourself the go-ahead to mend your relationships that may have been damaged along the way because of your addiction. Forgiveness of oneself also encourages positive thinking, and it may provide you with a sense of hope for your future. When you no longer have a figurative cloud of self-hatred or disdain hanging over your head, you are more likely to see a positive way out of your addiction. While every aspect of this process for understanding is important, it all begins with the ability to forgive, to let that negative view of yourself become dim, and replaced with a triumphant, confident, absolved self image.

GRATITUDE

Gratitude is a feeling of thanks and appreciation for benefits received, and for life in general. One of the best things you can do for yourself is to express gratitude for the little things. For example, if you were addicted to a substance of some form, you can be grateful for the fact that you still have your life. Far too many people die from various overdoses of different substances. Gratitude is the key to inner peace. When you constantly express gratitude for even the littlest of things, the universe will send you more things to be grateful for.

When there is an element of dependency in your life, it is difficult to be truly thankful. The primary focus is survival, whether that is through avoiding consequences or the attaining of your addiction fulfillment. Only then are you grateful, and it is a fleeting moment, replaced quickly by a ticking clock for when you will need to survive all over again. You tend to experience relief more than actual gratitude, to be honest. That is another excellent reason why this particular aspect is one that has possibly been forgotten, or simply gone unused.

Gratitude makes you more positive and open to new opportunities and lifestyles which will be beneficial to you. Grateful feelings for how far you have come from your past to your present affects you and those around you. Your energy becomes more positive when you are grateful; it even tells on your environment. There is true joy in being able to feel truly grateful for what you have, rather than simply being content with making it to the end of the day.

Take a deep breath and look around right now. Take stock of what is around you and what it reminds you of. What reminder of gratitude stuck out to you first? Were there more than one? There is rarely a bad time to pause and remind yourself about everything you can be grateful for. In fact, it often provides you with that clear perspective all over again, a good way to reflect on the positive changes that have been made, and the people by your side throughout.

By resolving your past, you are telling yourself that it is okay to move on to greener pastures. It is okay to forgive yourself for your past and live a life free of addiction. It is okay to be grateful for the little changes that have had a positive effect on your life. When you accept your past, you bring yourself closer to a positive present, and away from the past. By being in the present, we deal with the truth of our reality. The present lets us know where we are in our progress, and we can assess ourselves to determine what we need to do to live better lives. In being present, we can make use of the numerous resources that are available for people struggling with various types of addiction. These resources aid in recovery from whatever addiction you struggle with. There are specific apps for people in recovery, most of which are free. These apps provide people with addiction treatment and resources for recovery. Because they are mobile apps, it becomes easier and more convenient to keep track of your recovery by monitoring your triggers, keeping a virtual journal, and connecting with people who are also on the journey to recovery from addiction.

Aside from mobile apps, there are more conventional resources that you can use. There are self-help groups and 12-step recovery groups that can be of great help to you and your journey to recovery. Also, there are government websites that you can consult to find qualified and accredited addiction treatment programs. Addiction-recovery organizations such as the American Lung Association and the United Kingdom's Institute of Alcohol Studies play crucial roles in your road to recovery.

One cannot move forward in life without having confronted one's past. Running away from your past without dealing with it would prove detrimental in the future. It may even cause you to relapse. It is dangerous to leave your past unaddressed as doing so would make it a permanent fixture that promises to darken your life at unpredictable times. You should also ensure that you do not remain in one position, even after your recovery. Having gone through acceptance, forgiveness, and gratitude, your next step is to redirect your focus toward building a new life.

The best way to ensure that you move forward in life is by taking things one at a time and doing things at your own pace. Do not rush into your new life, or think that you are doing worse than other people because they seem to have recovered faster and better than you have. It is your journey so you should not compare the steps you take to anyone else's journey. Ensure that you live – truly – and take each day one at a time.

GENERAL POINTS FOR REVIEW

- Addiction is a byproduct of unaddressed trauma and emotional pain.
- You need to properly, deeply understand your past if you want to heal.
- What does it mean to heal?

- Healing is overcoming and restoring oneself to wellness.
- Steps to resolving your past:
- Acceptance
- Rid yourself of the "victim mentality."
- It is vital to recognize your pattern.
- Reassess your thinking as to where blame is placed.
- Forgiveness
- Forgiving yourself is just as important as forgiving others.
- The ability to forgive is a character trait that more people should strive for.
- Forgiveness is beneficial to you and to those you love.
- Gratitude
- What reminder of gratitude sticks out to you in your life?
- By resolving your past, you are telling yourself it is okay to move on.
- One cannot move forward in life without having confronted one's past.

4

A BALANCED AND PURPOSEFUL LIFE IS A SOBER LIFE

Imagine this scenario: You have a stable life, comfortable finances, fulfilling relationships, and goals and hopes for the future. One day, through no fault of your own, you are in an accident of some sort. In the time following this accident, you had to attend physical rehabilitation and were put on a prescription to help manage the considerable pain the injury was causing you. Most nerve injuries have a tendency to linger when it comes to pain, and can be predominant even when the physical rehab is working.

You had never experienced trauma to this extent before, and considering the sudden halt to your normal routine, you feel off balance. Your stress levels began to drastically increase, and with that came the added difficulty of working through both the physical and emotional damage. As you continue with your recovery, you run out of your Paid Time Off, and quickly run through the remaining Vacation Time you have at your place of work. Your boss tries to be understanding, but after the lengthy time off he cannot hold your position any longer and you are let go from your job.

Now the stress rises exponentially as you must still continue to heal, but the challenges continue to mount. Throughout this time you have begun to discover that the only time you find a semblance of peace is when you are taking your pain medication. A shift occurs in your mind and rather than seeing that medication as a physical remedy, it is now a way to find solace from the rapidly deteriorating structure of your life. You find yourself using a few more pills than usual during the day, but you are still okay is what you tell yourself.

The financial burden continues as your insurance runs out now that you are out of work. You were smart with money so you have savings, but now you have gone through your first prescription, and you are increasingly aware of how many pills you have remaining, plus the refills you are being allowed. You haven't gone out as much, or nearly at all lately, and your friends have started to notice and are mentioning their concern.

Something in the back of your mind is aware that the way you are handling your medication is not healthy, but the thought of not having a respite from the stress causes those thoughts to be stifled quickly. More calls from your friends, more dodging and making excuses. It seems each time you do this avoidance dance with your social circle, you have to take more medication to mask the rising realization that you are on a dangerous path.

Fast forward another month. You are out of prescription refills and are painfully aware of how many pills are in the last bottle. You haven't answered the phone in three days other than to try and convince your doctor to cut you a break with another refill. You know that everything is crumbling, but as long as you don't have to see it, you are okay. Your savings will last another few months, but you are becoming more worried because you aren't as worried about the money as you are with the pill situation.

Another few months go by and you no longer recognize yourself. Every routine you had is gone and now replaced with a grim survival mode. Nothing is in balance, and each day is a dismal stretch of hours leading to sleep. You still aren't quite sure how you got here, but you know it isn't right.

This story is heard often about how easy it is for a life to unravel when imbalance goes unrecognized. While yes, the presence of medication and circumstance provided a welcoming environment for addiction, it truly takes hold when you begin to ignore the changes in priority around you. This chapter will cover the damages that living a life without balance can cause, as well as how important it is to be aware of these imbalances.

The choice to move forward in a life of sobriety is an incredibly hard decision to make, but what proves to be even more difficult is living a life of imbalance. In order to maintain a cycle of addiction, it becomes an absolute necessity to live a double life. Neither face is genuine and are both equally false. This lack of balance leads to the cornucopia of issues and deterrents to sobriety we had gone over in the previous chapters: anxiety, depression, and eventually a path towards even more back and forth between those two faces. Make no mistake, you have both the strength and fortitude to correct this imbalance, but it takes a committed combination of faith and time.

Take a moment and consider what areas of your life endured the most disruption due to your addiction? While most people see a general deterioration in areas of their life, there is usually a primary place where they are impacted in a somewhat disproportionate manner. It may be unpleasant to think back to those times and circumstances, but it is a necessary challenge. It is not enough to simply *know* there were areas of imbalance, you must identify to the best of your ability *what* those areas were.

Perhaps you became extremely isolated and that social hermitage began the chain reaction to the other aspects of your life. Or maybe you were able to keep a false stability across everything except for in your marriage, and subsequently all the fallout from the rest of your life was funneled into the dysfunction brought to that relationship.

The details will differ as you discover the specifics, but it is worth setting the book down for a few minutes and really thinking it over.

Just as the lack of balance creates disruptions throughout your life, having balance and maintaining that aspect of your routine leads to increased peace and an atmosphere that promotes healing. There is transparency in a life of balance, an open policy with yourself about where your focuses lie, and why you choose to prioritize as you do. Across the scope of your daily life, you have different obligations and desires for how your time is being spent, and with each choice, you create your priority list. By recognizing these moments, you will have a clearer picture of where your time goes, and if there are imbalances, they are there to be addressed.

If you find yourself at the gym more than anywhere else and your choices in other circles of life begin to rely solely on your working out, that is an indicator of a priority that may need a closer look. There is nothing wrong with having work be a priority unless issues arise that deeply affect your family and personal life. A focal point for you, something that seems singular, may be an indicator of a different way that balance can impact a life, especially when in or with addiction. Addressing this is not a moment of judgment, because even on days where things may seem to lean a certain way, it does not always mean there is an imbalance. The presentation of a new routine carved out by a singular focus on one part of your life, however, is where the scales begin to tip in a direction that could indicate an addiction.

By breaking aspects of life down into concrete, readable portions, it gives a chance to breathe and take in the information. Over the next few sections, you will be able to see different areas where singular priorities could have a negative impact on your life. When appropriately balanced and committed to positive change, these areas combined form a healthy, forward-progressing approach to living.

Health and Fitness[1] [2]

The path to sobriety runs hand-in-hand with maintaining a healthy lifestyle. The actions themselves are as essential as creating and having a schedule that provides structure. Exercise does not have to be complicated; simply, the presence of consistency will help form those positive habits. When going through the recovery process, some activities are correctly used to help build those foundations. These are VACI's, or Vitally Absorbing Creative Interests, as SMART Recovery defines them; exercising, crafts, nature watching, all of these are excellent examples that all aid in rediscovering what used to bring joy rather than merely replacing those activities - the type that got to the point where you had to be using to enjoy them, or that directly influenced your addiction.

Research has shown that it is just *doing* the activity that can bring benefits. Something as easy as walking for thirty minutes a day is beneficial. It isn't only the physical aspect of this that cultivates an atmosphere of healing and growth. By having pre-planned activities scheduled, you won't simply justify not going out, or not disrupting that. Simple self-talk can help, "If I have to get up and run in the morning, I can't go out tonight where I could get a drink." Other small statements of the same nature can assist in those moments of persuasion.

For many people, not just those who struggle with addiction, there has never really been an interest in exercising. Despite the fact that it is commonly known to positively impact practically every aspect of your life, we still distance ourselves from it. If you took an isolated route during your addiction, there is a good chance you did not have a dedicated exercise routine. The same can be said for those whose addiction made working out particularly difficult. The specifics of why aren't the point, but rather that it may require a shift in perspective. This may not be an interest you enjoy, per se, but rather one that is purely here to provide stability and longevity.

You have made it through truly monumental struggles that many have not been able to; that is no small feat. Keeping that at the forefront of your mind, you should have a desire to do everything in your power to keep this newfound life intact and functioning. You've earned this chance, and including a physical aspect will be beneficial in many ways you may have not considered. Some of those benefits include elevated mood, better sleep patterns, increased positive energy, a healthy distraction, lower stress, and improvement to your overall well being[3]. What others have you experienced or can you think of?

There are other aspects of exercise, not physical, that can be beneficial to the process. One common issue that those in recovery encounter is that they have much more free time than they had previously. Periods through the day or week filled by that addiction are now gaps of unscheduled, stagnant time. Adding exercise to the schedule is a catalyst more than merely a time-filler; the workout itself is rarely the focal point.

Depending on the type of addiction, your body has been put through various situations and endured more than it was intended to. Because of this, there are levels and variations of healing that must occur. While the physical portion of exercising may not always be the focus, it is a massive boost to that healing process. Balancing hormones that hadn't been released accordingly, increased nerve connections in the brain, and laying a foundation for a more balanced sleep schedule stem from the physical healing gleaned during working out.

The world of exercise is expansive and sometimes complex for someone who has never really delved into that realm. To avoid disruption to your momentum, or any doubt in yourself, here are some examples of recommended workout routines specifically for those in recovery[4]:

- **Walking**: Especially early on in your recovery, you may not have a lot of energy. Withdrawals are also especially tiring, so this can be a good use of your time as well as getting some form of physical exercise in. Never discount the benefits of a brisk, thirty minute stroll.

- **Hiking:** This could be a gentle step up from the walking routine. Aim for the environment rather than the physical exertion. Being out in nature for extended periods of time has proven to have a plethora of benefits, ranging from physical to emotional. If you are an enthusiast, then feel free to go full pace with your equipment and effort but you should feel no obligation to do anything other than a mildly challenging, nature-based walk.
- **Yoga:** You would be hard pressed to find a group that discounted the positive effects of doing yoga. From increased breathing awareness to flexibility, the opportunities for bettering yourself can all have a firm anchor in the calm that yoga can bring. The varieties are growing every day, and thanks to its recent popularity, it is easy to find a local center that hosts classes. If the social aspect is intimidating, YouTube has an excellent library to choose from, all from the comfort and non-judgemental eyes of your own home.
- **Swimming**: While this may not always be the most convenient form of exercise, there is no denying the overall workout obtained from a mere twenty minutes in the pool. The main benefit is that it is a very low impact exercise, in case soreness or aches are particularly bad that day. As with the other exercises and suggestions in this section, you should feel no obligation to join a class or even do anything in an organized manner. Having the water around you and just floating can be exactly what you need.
- **Dancing:** Here is one of the more unorthodox suggestions, because it is often overlooked. A reason that people choose this over other forms of exercise is because it doesn't really *feel* like you are working out. There is an inherent aspect of fun that may not always be present in other methods you

have tried, or were considering. Another incentive is that many dance studios offer a first class for free, or at least a trial bargain. This has the potential to be a low-risk, fun, healthy, and social activity to give a try!
- **Team Sports:** While not as simple to be a part of, this may be a more relatable form of working out for those who had some sports influence in their life. Again, there are many variations of activity, along with different levels of skill and experience. You should never feel like you are overextending yourself with the addition of exercise, and when considering an organized team sport this should be a point of thought.

Team sports could also be an avenue to discovering something new! While the popular sports are well known, maybe do a little research and find a sport you never really gave consideration to before. Curling, badminton, or cricket are just a few examples of some less common variations you could try. You never know until you give it a shot.

- **Weight Lifting:** Finally, this is a more structured, typical approach to working out. While it is common and most gyms or workout rooms tend to have some form of weights, proceed with caution. Unless you are under supervision or have prior training, do not push yourself when it comes to weight training. While the basic act is simple, the potential for injury by taking on too much is a risk that you need to be aware of.

With these examples, hopefully you now have a better idea of ways to incorporate exercise into your schedule as a regular occurrence.

Spirituality[5]

Every person differs in their belief systems and how they view the concept of a higher power. Regardless of the differences between religions, the ability to turn to something larger than themselves plays a significant role in gaining and maintaining stability and balance. No matter the specifics of what you believe, there is a consistency when it comes to finding the power within. That place inside yourself, somewhere to turn to in daily meditation, is a healthy step in learning *how* to heal, and not only allowing it to happen.

The basis of spirituality is faith. Not only religion but faith in yourself, that circumstances can change, that belief in hope. Cultivating this creates a nurturing environment for a positive self-image to take root. So often in recovery, there is negativity in every version of self one can have, and this becomes both exhausting and deteriorates that gleam of hope.

Where exercise can impact mental health and is completed through action, faith has the ability to heal both the mind and body. The belief that there is value in who you are as a person is an invaluable characteristic to build, and this is begun deep within yourself. Where this aspect applies during the recovery process is a personal journey, but never forget that your strength of spirit can and will bring healing.

In a recent study by Adi Jaffe, PhD[6], he broke down the approach to spirituality while in recovery as being between two main camps of thought when it came to this subject. It was the Religious group and the Spiritual group, and while both have positive messages and can be essential for certain people to their success in recovery, both are vastly different.

Those from the Religious group tend to recognize a deity in some form, usually in a structure or order. The people who subscribe to this belief consider it necessary to commune in fellowship with those of a similar system and ideologies. This is where the Spiritual group differs. Having spiritual qualities does not directly infer the presence of a greater being, but is more of an unseen connection among all of us, a cosmic understanding and bond, of sorts.

While there are obvious differences between the two, they can converge on several key aspects in a healthy life free from dependency. Both schools of thought have variations of focus on returning a purpose to your life. They also believe in being a contributing member of society and the world - the order differs depending on the specifics. Along with these, the overarching idea that both camps agree on is finding something greater than yourself to believe in and use as a basis for faith.

Religion finds that in a god, or multiple gods, whereas Spirituality focuses on the belief that by coming together as a society, the best of ourselves, that real change can be affected; both within ourselves, and for the world.

Social Life[7]

During a discussion with a friend some time ago, the cutting of ties while in recovery came up. It is a commonly accepted truth that with the admittance of addiction and the subsequent recovery process, there will be a circle of friends with whom you will no longer socialize. This is usually considered one of the hardest steps to finding healing and peace through recovery. There would be unconditional acceptance across the board in an ideal world, and minimal changes would need to occur if any. Sadly that is not the case. As common as that is, it is just as common for that social gap to remain unaddressed.

There may arise the need to replace friends or that fewer friends directly correlate to lessened value. You lose no value when you choose your health over specific friends because while you cannot change the choices they make, you can distance yourself from a potentially toxic environment. This is not an easy decision but you must understand the power within it. You are giving yourself back the power in your life, and there are truths that go with attaining a healthy balance in your social realms.

One aspect that is certainly a truth and yet is rarely considered during the process is that things *will* change. While there may be some people you associate with that will be accepting of your choices and direction in life, many will not react how you may have expected at all. If you are not prepared for this then any balance across the other components of your life runs a risk of becoming unstable.

Do not discount the importance of this aspect. As we explained at the beginning of this chapter, isolation is an extreme detriment to your well being. This is one of the earlier red flags to be aware of, but it is also important to keep in mind as you are now rebuilding both yourself and your life. Yes, there may be relationships and areas that simply cannot be fully repaired, but you knew that real life consequences would occur. What you *can* do is find resolve to use that mistake, as with the others in your past, as a catalyst, an inspiration, to always be better; to always move forward.

Romantic Life[8][9]

Within recovery, it is commonly known that the maintenance of yourself and your sobriety is fragile in the early days, and could continue to be well into the process. It is because of that fragility that dating and any romantic endeavors are put out of mind until one year has passed. This alone can be a subject of contention and has been debated from multiple views over the decades, but what benefits to balance are there from waiting?

First, understand that this period of waiting is not any reflection of value or saying that you shouldn't have rewards from the new life of sobriety. This a moment you have worked hard for so, of course, you should be able to fully experience this fresh side of life. By not giving this the proper respect, because your sobriety is a serious matter, there is a risk that either priorities or perspectives could be skewed. It all comes back to balance and this particular subject is one that has more of a tendency than most to create that imbalance.

It is a natural characteristic within humanity to steer in the direction where the heart directs. It is a driving, strong force, one that begins to increase when a relationship begins to form. That type of connection brings with it a mass of complications that are difficult to maneuver in any circumstance, let alone for one beginning to learn balance within recovery. The desire to please and fulfill one's partner can be a powerful pressure to backslide into common patterns. It isn't merely the possible experiences while in a relationship, there is a real chance for disruption to your balance if these relationships end.

Throughout this process there will undoubtedly be times when you feel judged, attacked, pointed out, or that all the guidelines and expectations are unrealistic. Every one of those concerns is valid and should be considered extensively during your recovery. Relationships and romance can be a great boon or a disastrous journey no matter your past. Just like you had to admit your addiction, you must come to terms with what the recovery process is like and what future disruptions could occur.

Your health and your sobriety are always a singular focus. Find balance within that and romance, and all the ups and downs that go with it, shall come in time.

Hobbies

While in recovery there are two types of hobbies that you can undertake: productive ones and those for leisure. These two can intersect for certain activities, but most that you choose will fall under one of those two categories. Both are crucial to the process as they provide stimulation and are an excellent use of your "swap time," or time you used to devote to recovering from your addiction.

Hobbies are an excellent use of time, and they provide necessary distractions to curb the cravings. There is no need to feel pressured into picking up hobbies you have no interest in simply to *have* them. Taking enjoyment in the activities you choose is crucial to maintaining that overall balance in your life. One of the first, and most important steps you took on this journey was admitting the addiction, and with that comes the acceptance that the road *will* be difficult, that cravings will happen. The structure of these hobbies is a healthy way to alleviate the weight of those times, in addition to creating that foundation of stability.

Just as we discussed with exercise and working out in general, your skill level has nothing to do with the activity or hobby. You may not be training for the Olympics, but your effort and time spent will result in benefits to both your health and path of sobriety.

Career

This can be a touchy subject for certain people depending mainly on how your addiction impacted your work. Some addicts maintained a stable work life and let the imbalances fall to the other sectors of their lives; many others saw a direct and negative effect at their place of work and on the quality overall. It is precisely because of these reasons, and that is a trigger subject, that it must be addressed.

No matter the program you are in for recovery, there is a section or step regarding work and careers. It is a part of life in general to not only seek out work, but to find one that fulfills and rewards. That does not change due to your recovery, in fact you may find that your work life has *more* meaning. As with your personal life, you had to either hide or work your addiction into your routine to avoid being found out. This is an exhausting cycle and the burden alone brings with it anxiety, stress, and directly impacts your performance on the job. Stepping forward in this new, refreshed life will feel new and situations that had brought paranoia or triggered your addiction can now be stepping stones and reminders of the changes you have made, and are continuing to make.

A career can also be an excellent goal to work towards. Depending on your past, furthering yourself at work may not have been an option due to either substances or time needed for your secrets. A brand new road is before you now, and with that comes increased advancement opportunities if you stay the course. When those difficult moments arise you will have a concrete reason to push through without giving in!

Be prepared for the moments that trigger your addiction, especially in the workplace. In a perfect world, the transition would be easy and every situation would be ideal without the hint of temptation, but you know full well this will not be the case. Even under the best of circumstances you will still encounter those moments from time to time, but that does not reduce their importance. You are going to have more time on your hands and you will be aware of these times. When a cigarette smoker decides to quit they will no longer take smoke breaks. Suddenly they are painfully aware of the 5-10 minute periods they used to have, particularly if those breaks were based on a schedule. A coworker in a previous job told me that, for him, the hardest times were thirty to forty-five minutes after he got to work, and after meals. By identifying those specific times to expect the cravings to hit he gave himself the chance to be prepared. Applying these methods to your workplace is telling yourself that you have value, enough to put thought into things of this nature.

While every aspect of balance we covered can be individually applied to your journey, they are all moving you towards a bigger picture. Early in your sobriety these are used to create a foundation, something to build from towards your brighter future. These experimentations of pursuits are moving pieces that navigate you to your purpose. That is what it all boils down to: what will your impact on this world be?

Your life has both meaning and purpose. Addiction caused a temporary disruption of your road towards that goal, but it in no way destroyed it. Patience is key in this process, and by allowing every step and progression to arrive in its own time you are allowing yourself the vulnerability to accept it when you are ready. Outside of yourself there is no one who can tell you your calling, but when it happens it will feel right.

Don't fight this feeling when it occurs. Sometimes our past can make us hesitant to accept rewards or positivity because there is a part that feels we do not deserve it. That somehow by sacrificing good things we can help make up for mistakes and negative actions committed. This is a misguided reaction, though a very relatable sentiment. You will be working to uphold your sobriety for the rest of your life, you do not need to cause yourself grief to satisfy guilt. Instead, find closure and solace in the joy from furthering this new life you fought to regain.

Discovering your purpose has little to do with you and more to do with the effect you will have going forward; that is precisely how you know it is your purpose. A selfless instinct takes over and it is about the work, bettering humanity and everything around us. It is important to remember this because too often we are searching so hard that we search right past our path. There is a fluidity to this process; a flexibility to let things happen and move forward in the steps you know to follow. Everything starts somewhere, and keeping these guidelines in mind will give you direction when things get tough - and they will, but you are tougher. Much tougher.

Your past is exactly that and is behind you now. The issues have been addressed and you are in a forward motion. Part of this is accepting that your present is allowed to be rewarding and success is something you are deserving of. Living with an intentional balance and in a purpose-driven way makes sobriety a pretty straight forward path. This is not to say that it isn't fraught with obstacles, but with the keys you have learned the path forward is clearer.

Regarding these obstacles you have been given a checklist of your own design as we've moved through this chapter. The aspects of balance - *Health and Fitness, Spirituality, Social Life, Romantic Life, Hobbies,* and *Career* - provide something to reflect back upon if you recognize a pattern emerging that could lead to relapse, even early signs. Going through your balance keys will give you a better view of what is causing this disruption to your progress. There is no room for judgement here, in fact you should be praised for putting effort into ensuring your success in a sober life. Losing balance creates that sense of instability that can trigger an episode of engaging in vices.

You have value and worth. From that you are worthy of patience, from others and from yourself. Everything learned here is put in place for the benefit of anyone who is willing to commit not just to a new life, but a balanced approach to that lifestyle. It is with all this in mind that the next part of the journey begins. Patience is needed throughout the balancing process, as it is needed when you begin forming new, healthy habits. This is what we will cover in the next chapter.

GENERAL POINTS FOR REVIEW

- The lack of balance leads to a cornucopia of issues and deterrents to sobriety.
- What areas of your life endured the most disruption due to your addiction?
- By breaking down aspects of life, it gives a chance to take in the information.
- Keys to Balance:
- Health and Fitness
- Walking
- Hiking
- Yoga
- Swimming
- Dancing
- Team Sports
- Weight Lifting
- Spirituality

- Social Life
- Romantic Life
- Hobbies
- Career
- Your life has both meaning and purpose.
- Going through your Keys to Balance will give you a better view of what is causing disruptions to your progress.

5

DEVELOPING NEW HABITS

The life of one in recovery is a life of habits, whether these habits brought you to your addiction or those that you are forming now to heal from those decisions. As you no doubt know, some habits form easily and smoothly fit into our lives. Others, more commonly, take dedication and time to build up.

Now that you have begun to reverse those old, destructive habits, you can move forward in confidence towards starting new ones. Everything has an origin, and the creation of these positive new habits begins with simple, daily choices. This is going to be a slow process, one that will require small steps, truly walking before you run. In no way is this a race and haste will not serve you well on this journey. Take comfort in this fact. It is a rare thing indeed in this life to have a reason to slow down and think, plan, and *then* act. Depending on your type of addiction you may have experienced the pace much faster than you were comfortable with; this is a gift, not just the opportunity that recovery presents, but that you have the time to take this at a healthy, steady pace.

There are several reasons that defy common sense showing that forming these new, positive habits are beneficial to the new leaf you are turning over. As discussed previously, having time on your hands during this phase in your life is certainly inadvisable, if not directly harmful, and you know that this free time is an inevitability as a side effect of your sobriety. These habits take that time and put it to a good use; thirty days to build a habit, we've heard this, and that is one month that you will be putting time and effort into this work.

Take a moment to think about what habits that you either have or are planning to begin as part of healthy routines. Just as the process of creating habits takes time, so does the process as a whole. Allowing yourself the freedom to pause and absorb when needed is going to be crucial to avoid feeling overwhelmed.

A large part of recovery is understanding that you are not alone with the struggle, not alone with the urges, and certainly not alone with the human weaknesses we all must battle. It is in these times that being self-aware becomes important. Without that awareness, the feeling of being alone can evolve into something much more dangerous to your health and well being. Going from feeling alone to a spiral is too close a connection to risk over simply not noticing. Being here, fighting to regain your life, signifies that you are *much* stronger than that.

Along with being aware of letting feelings become a road to regression, it is vital to be aware of old patterns that could emerge during times of difficulty. Before recovery, your usual reaction to an obstacle or hardship was to turn to your addiction, or at the very least begin conducting yourself in ways that will lead directly to it. Recognizing the formation of these old, negative habits will go a long way towards avoiding them.

A good definition for these negative habits is *a patterned behavior regarded as detrimental to one's physical or mental health*[1]. The key word there is "pattern," and for those in recovery, this can be a trigger word but it is certainly relatable. Just understanding that it *may* happen is not enough, you must identify what brings about those cycles of destruction. There are many variables that come into account when discussing the catalysts for these patterns, so let's look over a few[2].

- **Observance can be key**. Notice changes in yourself, or your surroundings, that reflect behaviors leading to or directly correlating with your addiction.
- **Expecting immediate perfection**. Keep in mind that recovery aims to progress you to a place of peace and healing, not a fast track to a result.
- **Keeping old perspectives**. Even though you have made significant changes in your life, especially concerning your addiction, you may still have ways of thinking that became so common they are now instinct. "More is better," could be one, or "try anything once." The wording isn't the point, but rather the possibility of that thought process's destination.
- **Recovery in a rut**. Just as recovery is not a quick fix, there is no maximum timeline either. How long you are in the stages of recovery vary greatly from person to person. Feeling stuck or stagnant can be a path back towards old patterns.

These are just a few possible instances to be aware of. Perhaps you didn't relate to any of these. That is okay, and it gives you the opportunity to use your self awareness. Ask yourself what your variables are that could lead back to old patterns? It doesn't have to be a direct action or traumatic event, but rather, as in the list above, it could be a perspective shift or a thought process.

Just as the negative patterns and cycles of behavior can lead back to the life of addiction you left behind, there are positive reciprocals of those same patterns. By implementing these in your life you allow yourself the benefits that come from sober, healthy routines. These can be across a broad spectrum, and it is important to give yourself time to discover which ones work for you. If you got no joy whatsoever from flying kites, it most likely will not make for a good hobby. Not that it isn't a healthy, outdoor activity, but rather that you will give you no emotional benefit, and tension caused from not enjoying it can turn the situation into a negative experience.

You deserve to have hobbies and routines that you take pleasure in, as long as you recognize the responsibility you also have to your sobriety. So instead of kites, maybe you prefer watching documentaries, or playing chess. Whatever you end up deciding on, remember that you are not relegated to a single hobby. Keeping an open mind and an attitude of awareness will be a large help in this discovery of enjoyment.

There are aspects of this process that are rarely brought up for the public view. If your addiction involved a substance, no doubt it enhanced special activities or made mundane ones enjoyable. Perhaps your addiction itself was the enjoyable activity, or one that brought you the feeling you desired: overeating, self-harm, and the like. However you came across it, once you remove yourself from the addiction, you may find that activities lack interest of any kind. This is normal and with effort and time will begin to be rectified. Your body and mind had become used to relying on the chemical release from the addiction for the euphoric feeling, rather than an activity bringing it about in the intended biological fashion. So now you must retrain both your body *and* mind in how to release those chemicals correctly. You are fully capable and empowered to achieve this, and excel while doing it! Patience, effort, and you make the unbeatable team that has already come so far. Imagine how far you can go!

Take a moment to think about what positive habits you have picked up since you started this new, fresh journey. There is a very good chance that you have put something healthy into motion without even realizing you were establishing a new pattern. Here are some possible options that you could consider, or maybe to add to those that you already are doing:

- **Cleaning.** Chores around the house, dusting, polishing can be both productive and healthy. If repetition is a positive tool for you, consider this as a good habit replacement.
- **Communication.** Isolation is a massive red flag, and has probably been an aspect of your life during your addiction. By reaching out more often than you used to, you allow for transparency to be cultivated. Family and friends, especially those who are familiar with your struggles, are excellent sources for support. A fun conversation is always a boost, as well.
- **Find peace.** Being mindful is a key factor in your journey. "Mindfulness is the basic human ability to be fully present, aware of where we are and what we're doing..."[3] Adjoining this mindset with the practice of meditation creates an atmosphere of growth, healing, and honesty with yourself. All of this translates to a better sense of self, better peace of mind, and a healthier step towards the life you are trying to create.
- **Exercising.** As we discussed before, do not be intimidated by the word *exercise*. You are not being asked to train for the Olympics - to train for anything, actually. Rather, it is the act itself, as minimal or intense as desired, that creates the new, healthy habits. Getting yourself into the pattern of being active in some way is an important variable of recovery. Do not be afraid to look for that one thing that piques your interest; yoga, Crossfit, or even just jogging a little. It all works, and it will all benefit you and your sober lifestyle!
- **Learn something new.** Depending on the places your addiction took you, there may have been many conversations at the peaks of the highs where elaborate plans were made to do such and such, and when the slope of the crash hit no actions were taken. This time is different, because *you* are different. Finding a new skill and putting the time and effort into learning it can be both satisfying and incredibly

therapeutic. The possibilities are vast, so take your pick with your triggers in mind.

- **Books or podcasts.** Both of these can be fruitful. Another factor to consider is attention span. If yours is particularly low, maybe try an audiobook rather than a physical book. You can still get the story, or the impact of the words, but you don't have to be singularly focused on it, which can often trigger anxiety and spirals if not handled correctly. The same goes with podcasts. Perhaps newspapers or magazines are not matching with your preferences, but you still want to have an intake of news and entertainment, or any subject you desire. By searching for and listening to a variety of podcasts, you will be taking positive action, but without stress and tension.
- **Cooking.** You are not aiming to become a Michelin-rated chef. This is about finding an interest that can help form new habits. By learning new recipes and techniques, you open yourself up to healthy avenues for your energy.
- **Diet.** This can go hand-in-hand with the cooking habit. By taking an active interest in your well being - and this includes the physical aspect, as well - you place value on yourself. Don't be afraid to try something new here, because you never know what could end up being an unexpected favorite!

All of this may seem like a great deal of information, and that is because it is. Starting fresh, especially in recovery, means retooling yourself for a world that you have most likely been avoiding for years. Simply because you feel overwhelmed does in no way mean you are underprepared. Expect to feel the struggle, but do not expect to give in to it.

Depending on the route you have taken, you may have had guidelines or suggestions made to you that require what could be considered "deleting" old habits and replacing them. It is important to not feel pressured into completely removing portions of yourself. The reasons you became addicted are usually directly linked to characteristics you possess. There is a tendency to steer yourself towards what interests you, or what could possibly enhance those interests. This does not simply mean making cartoons funnier or getting through long shifts without needing sleep, it also pertains to a desire for numbness, or to detach. These are interests as well, and you cannot discount their impact on how you make connections to activities or hobbies.

The reason that being asked to completely discard these connections seems so daunting is that the achievement is virtually impossible. This is not an issue of replacement, but rather of using that same energy and mindset to redirect your activities and time. Everything is done in steps, and this process is no different. Jumping in before preparation is taken into account will rarely result in something beneficial. Rather, begin by creating a space for these redirected patterns. This can be within your schedule or an actual, physical space in which to cultivate. Effort translates into increasing the value you recognize in an action. Because you are taking the time to create stability rather than rush to an immediate goal you are giving these new tools and what you have learned the chance to take root. Focus on each footstep along the way, not the destination you are heading towards.

It is important to remember that there are many different roads you can take on this fresh start to your life. There is no singular method, no sole process that leads to a sober utopia. Instead it is a matter of utilizing your self awareness and being mindful, quiet, and vulnerable in the present. One of these possible processes is a training technique called Habit Reversal Training[4].

This is a series of steps that help identify habits through awareness, and how to act in a more positive and healthy manner moving forward. You could consider this a form of impulse control, or a way to address damaging, consistent behavior. While we are going to unravel this process and break down the sections, remember that actually undergoing this type of therapy and intervention is done under observation and the responsibility of a trained professional. Not only that, but the conditions were closely monitored as well, ensuring that health and safety were the primary focus.

If this seems like something that will work for you, allow yourself the openness to unbiasedly view the series of actions and steps that make up this form of habit adjustment.

The actual implementation of the Habit Reversal Training is done by first Gaining Awareness, then Developing a Competing Response, Relaxation Training, Building Motivation, and finally Generalization. Every step is interconnected with the program as a whole; if, however, you find pieces and phrases that speak to you, hold those close and remember them. Simply because you cannot conduct this type of therapy on yourself does not mean you cannot gain something from learning about the applications.

Gaining Awareness

Without self awareness, you cannot hope to have a consistent, healthy, and sober life. By recognizing "destructive patterns," you are better prepared to identify them as they arise.

Developing a Competing Response

This is a rewording of a very specific form of replacing one habit with another. These can be large, sweeping adjustments, or small, detail-oriented changes.

Relaxation Training

Some people refer to the process of altering habits like this as a form of "self surgery." It isn't pretty, it usually hurts, but it is for your own good in the end. Because of this you *must* expect the struggles of anxiety, stress, and pushback from your own mind as you progress through this. Learning to relax and ease off the pressure will be vital in maintaining your will and energy throughout this process. By being able to have that relaxation ability, if a trigger presents itself you can respond in a healthy, calm manner.

Building Motivation

In this step, there is a combination of response techniques used to influence how motivation is utilized. Both negative and positive reinforcements are put into use to create balance. The positive aspect could be praise from those aware of your struggle and the process, while the negative could be the judgements you still see from people who haven't been able to forgive or let go yet. Both satisfy different aspects of the program and work together to help the formation of new habits.

Generalization

As the final step, this is where you learn how to transfer what you have learned into a real life setting. There is a major difference between learning a process and putting it into implementation. The responses you will get, and the reactions, will be guidelines to how the process is going and where adjustments may be needed.

This technique has been through trial-and-error studies since the 1970's, always under the consistent eye of both psychologists and neuroscientists. It is important to keep coming back to this point because the steps and process laid out in this book are for self-help, and while the topic of Habit Reversal has been covered, it is still a professional method.

Part of the process of creating these healthy habits is learning how to incorporate them into your routine. As a first step when out of recovery, the routine stands as a paramount aspect of this entire journey. Many times when those in your position go about trying to find interests to productively use their time, or simply to distract themselves from those cravings and pangs of addiction-related nostalgia, these attempts are met with obstacles. While "new" elicits a picture of something fresh and open, it can become problematic when looking at it from the perspective of assimilating this into your schedule.

Consider a change in perspective first, and putting things into practice second. Instead of seeing the new habits and your current routine as two separate entities that have to be somehow combined, look through a positive lens. Your routine is a functioning, changing creature, not a concrete, unmoving tablet of rules. As you learn and adjust to a sober life, your priorities will shift and the way you conduct yourself, and your time, will change accordingly. It is precisely because of these characteristics that introducing a new habit into your schedule is an organic process. There is no end-all method for doing this, and as such you must allow for trial-and-error. See where these new activities or interests of yours line up with how you allocate your time and go from there.

With this in mind, let's move forward into different ways you can incorporate the examples of positive habits we covered. Keep in mind the fluidity of your schedule and that you should be striving for flexibility, these pointers can help.

- Pick a time to wake up every morning that is conducive to your schedule, and stick to it. Use alarms or your partner helping or whatever can be a positive motivator to wake up at that time every day.
- Ensure time in your schedule for exercise. If you leave it to "when it happens" you are not cultivating structure.
- Meal planning can be a good, repetitive use of time that has productive results. This can work well into the cooking and diet aspects we covered before.
- Your well-being extends outside your mind and your physical self is a large part of it. Establish a self care routine that can help that same structure, but also one that will establish value within yourself.
- Household cleaning can be tedious, but when viewed from

the perspective of personal growth, it becomes a productive use of time. Consider creating a Chore Schedule to help put those habits into practice.

- A big part of self-care is hygiene. Depending on what path brought you here, that aspect may have suffered in the past. Seeing yourself as a person of value, and therefore worth the effort, is revelation in action.
- Finally, developing new skills is not only productive, it continues that trend of self worth. You may have lived from day to day in a survival mode, as many in recovery have. The future extended only for as long as the high, rush, or numbing lasted. Then everything was focused on continuing that feeling. You are on a different road now, a road of compassion and love towards yourself. By learning new things, big or small, you are telling yourself that there is a future to be worked towards. A future you want to be a part of.

These are guidelines and if you do not feel they mesh well into the sober lifestyle you are cultivating, then there is no harm in reading them and moving past. If, however, you feel a defensive reaction to any of these, then take a moment and explore that. Why would your first instinct be to go on the defensive? Maybe it was simply a knee jerk reaction relating to a past experience, and if so that can be addressed in itself. If the reason is because you feel attacked, that can be a signifier of something that needs exploratory if not invasive "self surgery." You are making these changes and implementing these actions for the betterment of your life and everyone you interact with. You can give yourself that few seconds to find the origin of your instinctual reaction.

You have been given a great deal of knowledge in this chapter alone, but the most important habit, one of positivity and progression, is that of Gratitude Reflection. This can take many forms - journaling, verbal pep talks, mindful focus - but the core principle is to create an atmosphere of gratitude and recognizing the moments that deserve that attention.

Journaling can be a key aspect of this and one that has the ability to keep the positive momentum going. Acknowledging these moments of thankfulness is not always enough. Our daily life is filled with interactions, conversations, thoughts, media, and countless other things that fill our minds. To expect that, on a daily basis, you can think back over the course of your day and pick out those key times when you noticed the need to be grateful is not realistic. Those are not just passing moments that get a nod, they are important and they matter much more than you may think. Keeping a journal doesn't have to be a line by line review of your day, nor does it have to be some ultra-personal confidante for secrets and whispers. It can simply be a Gratitude Journal. Its sole purpose is to document when these little bits of thankfulness crept in, and how often. That will provide you with a scrapbook of sorts to chart your journey.

Were there weeks where the pages seem a little blank? Or, on the other side, perhaps you notice a pattern where you had an overflow of these moments. By identifying them you can understand your reactions more, and see the world for the wondrous place it is.

Now, there are those of us who never took to keeping a journal. The reasons are not the important part, what *is* important is that not having that outlet creates the same issue as thinking you'll remember those significant moments. If journaling itself is not appealing, consider taking up meditation or schedule a daily, quiet, isolated time for yourself to reflect back on the day's events. Whatever the method, the importance is in the recognition of those moments of Gratitude Reflection.

The BAART Program (Bay Area Addiction Research and Treatment) has been serving the city and area of San Francisco since the 1970's[5]. From their expertise and knowledge came many different techniques and methods by which to treat many addictions, primarily those with an opioid history. Among these were five habits that would be foundational in creating stability within a sober life. Some of these touch on aspects we have covered, so the focus will be more generalized.

1. Eat a Healthy Diet
2. Add Exercise to Your Schedule
3. Practice Healthy Sleep Habits
4. Form Connections With Others
5. Nurture Your Interests[6]

As you can see, many of the programs and resources devoted to helping those who have chosen a sober path have similar bases in thinking. While ideologies and how to implement certain practices cause differences among these various programs and organizations, the fact remains that with the focus on your well being, your sobriety, and your future, you will have no trouble learning strength and how to continue your forward progress.

It is a mantra worth having: small steps, small steps. If you prefer quotes, then, "Rome wasn't built in a day." Regardless of the presentation, the truth remains the same. You are a person of value, and through that perspective, you can change the habits that were detrimental and build up positive, new habits that will encourage you to flourish. With patience and the correct view of your self worth, nothing is beyond your reach, especially stability and happiness in a future that is safe and healthy.

You are capable, you are strong. Never let those words slip your mind.

GENERAL POINTS FOR REVIEW

- The life of one in recovery is a life of habits.
- Now that you have begun to reverse old, destructive habits

- you can move forward in confidence.
- A negative habit is *a patterned behavior regarded as detrimental to one's physical or mental health.*
- What brings about your cycles of destruction?
- Observance can be key
- Expecting immediate perfection
- Keeping old perspectives
- Recovery in a rut
- Just as there are negative habits, there are positive, productive ones
- Possible healthy habits to consider:
- Cleaning
- Communication
- Find peace
- Exercising
- Learn something new
- Books or podcasts
- Cooking
- Diet
- Habit Reversal Therapy:
- Gaining awareness
- Developing a competent response
- Relaxation training
- Building motivation
- Generalization
- Have you tried journaling as an outlet/positive habit?
- Five foundational habits for creating stability (BAART Program):
- Eat a healthy diet
- Add exercise to your schedule
- Practice healthy sleep habits
- Form connections with others
- Nurture your interests
- "Rome wasn't built in a day."

6

STAYING ACTIVE TO MOVE FORWARD

Change is never easy; this you know very well, and we've covered how change can take a variety of forms. There is a saying, "The best revenge is a life well lived." This is applicable because a common reason that those in recovery struggle in finding fulfillment in their lives post-addiction is that they feel they need to be punished for what occurred. Every time they falter or stumble in their journey, it is seen as an inevitable consequence of living the way they had been. This is a myth that *must* be dispelled immediately. Your past is what it is, and the way you rectify the wrongs and ripples caused by it is between yourself, your sponsor, and your loved ones. Make no mistake, you do not deserve to punish yourself. What you *do* deserve is to cultivate a life that will give power to your sobriety. You deserve joy and success and this can only be done by first finding forgiveness from yourself.

This concept is difficult for those who have not experienced life in recovery. When work is put forth and rewards are given like promotions, bonuses, etc., it is very common for the sober employee or friend to feel they are not worthy of this recognition. The logic is that somehow, over time, the amount of times you sacrifice the chance for something good, you get closer to a moral balance. Do you find it hard to accept praise? If you have been promoted since you began your sober life, did you feel like you couldn't accept it or that you didn't deserve it? These are not uncommon reactions, and by utilizing your self-awareness, you can be more cognizant of when these situations occur. It takes willpower and strength to put those kind of instinctual reactions aside, it isn't easy, but you are fully capable of accomplishing this!

Once you are able to not only see yourself in a future, but have that future be one of success and positivity, you have taken a large step. The key term is *forward*. Stagnancy, as we've discussed, rarely breeds progress. Just as the steps you've taken up to now have put a focus on seeing value in yourself, seeing a future for yourself creates worth as well.

While you may struggle with aspects from your past for some time - which is normal, and should be expected - understand that it holds no power or sway in your life now. You will always associate certain thoughts or even lessons with things in your past, be it good or bad, but it is not a place you can dwell. There is a method sometimes used when handling extreme trauma in a time-sensitive situation: letting emotions in. What that means is to allow yourself a moment to truly feel what your mind and soul are experiencing be it grief, joy, guilt, or the other countless feelings you could have. You only allow it to exist for that moment, though. You are in control. This technique can also be used when you experience those feelings that make a healthy future seem out of reach or not deserved. These reactions are a direct result of guilt, and while they are not a true reflection of who you are now, they exist and are real. Because of this, but for only a few moments, feel it. Understand the depth of the emotion, and then take back control. This will not be easy the first time, or even over the course of time, but the repetition creates the signifier of importance. You have placed value on this and will therefore put in the necessary effort to attain it.

When it comes to control, has your past caused you to place limitations on your present self? This goes back to feeling the need to punish yourself for your past actions. Your present is something fresh and new that's not controlled by your past. Do not allow the stigma that has been placed on those in recovery to taint how you view your future. There is a judgement that can follow those who struggle with addiction, and it is not only incorrect but also damaging to the progress trying to be made.

You've explored new interests and allowed yourself to be vulnerable, and all of it is done in pursuit of creating a balanced life. It all comes back to balance, and remembering to keep yourself in check regarding this. Refer back to the list of aspects in your life that require attention, and how they are prioritized. When you feel "off" or like you may slip, take stock of how the balance in your life is. If you are truly honest with yourself, there is most likely some part of your life that isn't being given the priority it deserves. Life is life. That sounds redundant but, at the end of the day, it's a simple truth. No matter if you are in recovery, an athlete, a lawyer, unemployed, or any other walk of life, life is just that: *life*. Expect turbulence, expect the road to become cracked and difficult to traverse, expect to stumble. Once you accept those facts, you can be ready when they occur and prepared to correct any imbalance.

It requires humility to take those steps, and you have developed the tools to put that humility into practice. By moving forward with this attitude, you can be vulnerable in the face of a world that is harsh and unfeeling more often than not. Do not be disheartened in those moments, because it is very easy to be overwhelmed when your skin is thin. There is an inherent fragility that comes from a person being open and vulnerable; the knowledge is that such vulnerability may cause them harm, sometimes deep and lasting. Your well-being is well worth that effort, and as long as *you* are dedicated to both the process and the belief in yourself, the risk will result in reward.

Action. Nothing happens without it, and in its absence there is detriment and imbalance. There is a very good chance that at some point in your past you tried the "wait and see" technique of avoiding consequence and responsibility. If you were a student of this body of thought then you also know the results are negative, and usually to a much greater proportion than if you had taken action. You know the story well, I'll bet. Someone runs out of means to feed their addiction, so they engage in something illicit or illegal to obtain the resources. Once they are able to use, the fear of being without fades and any future consequence also drifts away in justifications. You knew full well that the wrong action you took to get you the substance or means will have a reciprocal response, and the longer it goes unaddressed, the greater the consequence grows exponentially. By the time the high wears away or the numbness melts to feeling again, you are left with a stark realization of what it took to get you there. You weren't ready to address the underlying addiction and undergo the necessary changes, and the only action you can think to take is no action whatsoever. If you wait, then at least you have the time until you're "found out" to enjoy calm.

From that point, everything begins to snowball. No doubt you have to act in more secrecy than usual because you assume everyone knows what you did. Still you remain silent, stoic, waiting it out. Early in your addiction, you most likely got away without consequence a few times and that created a sense of being untouchable, so you saw it as a viable option when faced with a crisis stemming from your addiction. Inaction followed by more of the same eventually creates an ugly, distorted result where the hurt is spread over multiple parties and the damage is sometimes beyond what even you imagined. Everything comes back to one thing: the decision not to act.

Your life did not magically turn itself around and start on a new, healthy path. It wasn't an accident; you did this. You made a conscious decision to take action, going against every instinct you had built during your addiction. This same ideology applies through the remainder of your journey. Every day, you have to make that choice all over again. Routine, as we covered earlier, is a critical part of a balanced life, and including that choice into your schedule makes it all the more real. Say it loudly, repeat it as many times as you need to because when your health, future, and well being are at stake, there isn't room for feeling silly or judged. Never accept anything less from yourself than the courage that brought you here. Take action every time, especially when it seems like the most difficult thing to do.

Your life is a byproduct of the actions you take. The mistakes in your past are linked to a lack of action as equally as the times you decided to continue in your addiction. Creating an environment where you can string together a series of positive actions will continue that healthy cultivation of self you have been striving for. Keep it in the back of your mind, the forefront, and on the tip of your tongue at all times. *Take action!* Take action for yourself, for those you love who support you, and because your future is worth it. *You* are worth it.

Just as inaction can be detrimental to your success in a sober life, a lack of goals will also impact how you progress towards the future. Earlier it was explained how in your past you lived without a future; survival was the singular focus and anything else was trivial. The difference is that now survival depends on your positive choices rather than in enabling an addiction.

When you look ahead in life, far down the road, what do you see? Have you considered it? How far ahead do your plans go? Maybe you have a 5-year plan, or maybe you are still learning how to expand your thinking from a day-to-day agenda to something with longevity. However you are going about it, the point is to have your eyes set on goals, both short- and long-term. This is not only to ensure you are prepared for what is to come, but also because stagnancy takes many forms. A lack of vision for the future is often overlooked.

When those in recovery recount experiences, some of the keywords used are *haze* or *blur*. That is the entire point, really, in feeding that addiction. When the concept of time becomes based on a series of highs and lows it will feel chaotic, unkempt, and out of your control. The point is that you gave up your control of your own time to your addiction, and now is the time to take it back.

Why is having goals so imperative to this process? To living a healthy, sober life? It gives you back ownership of your time. You can schedule and plan weeks, months, and even years to attain the goals you set before you. Don't hesitate to make multiple variations as well. Have specific short term goals, have those that you wish to accomplish within 5-10 years, and then give yourself the freedom to imagine the apex of your success. Where is that place for you? By identifying that dream, that goal, you give power to it. It is no longer just a quiet desire in your mind; it is alive on paper or in text in front of you. Keep this list of goals close to you, no matter how short or long your list is. Folded in your pocket, written on your phone or computer, the medium isn't the point. The point is simply having it on hand as a reminder in difficult moments. Don't be afraid to look it over whenever you feel unbalanced or off your usual routine. Give yourself back ownership of time that is truly *yours*.

When the idea of time comes up, you must also prepare yourself for when your addiction tries to regain control of you and ownership of your time with it. It isn't a violent grab either, this you know all too well. It is a gentle coaxing, a caressing and reassurance that this is the right way to go. That you "deserve to feel good." In response to that in particular, you *do* deserve to feel good and on *your* own terms, not the addiction's terms. Until you find that balanced point and understand the awareness of self needed, then implement it in your life, you have to be ready for when those gaps in your time give way to those creeping thoughts. In those moments, the early time on this journey is when you will build the foundation that your future can be built on. It is a base of personal strength, willpower, and taking back control over both your goals and your time.

Once you view your future as attainable, and understand how to own your time, you can make the push forward towards that unfolding life. You are not simply going through the motions of recovery, your goals are real and are *yours*. You must come at this from the perspective that your goals and the steps to them are not solely part of a plan to prevent a relapse. There is a much bigger, much more important picture going on and it has you at the center.

Throughout this journey you have been building towards the goal of a well balanced, healthy, sober life. In order to achieve this, a plan has been formulating, created from the guidelines and lessons you have picked up along the way. It is vital to have that plan, that preparedness, when you are working towards the future you desire. That includes benchmarks as you reach certain points in this growth.

As with any program designed to enhance your personal growth, the two main types of goals are broken down into short- and long-term. Both are important to the final result, just as they are equally substantial towards maintaining. People learn and are rewarded in different ways, and the attention to that individuality means being aware of how you respond as well. Do you know in what way you are best rewarded to stay motivated?

Are you long-term oriented? Primarily focused on what will happen down the road, and the larger, more time-intense goals act as a motivator? People who have these tendencies are less inclined to see the more immediate, small-reward goals as a catalyst; they instead see these short-term goals as more of a distraction, or even an inconvenience. If this sounds like you, gear your sights towards those larger, big picture destinations; trying to force a system on yourself that is not efficient for you has no benefits.

Now, maybe you are motivated by those short-term goals, and that is perfectly fine as well. Without knowing your individual preferences and what best propels you forward, you will not be getting the most out of the processes you undertake. Focus on the smaller goals, the "stepping stone" goals. You won't be cannon-balled out of the water by the concrete results, but the practical applications and how they make you feel will be more fulfilling than if you made yourself wait for a reward that made the journey there less impactful.

Your well being and health are at stake, so ignore all those outside voices and listen to your own self: what form of learning speaks to you? How will you be motivated best to stay the course? *Those* are the real, important questions to be asking. Luckily, the answers are just as important.

A significant term was used previously, and used often, throughout this book. That word is *guideline*. The reason that this specific expression is used is that you should always refer to experts when it comes to concrete, practical advice. While every technique and lesson has been created to better serve your sobriety and teach you how to best prepare for the long haul of a healthy, refreshed life, it is not medically certified. In short, this is **NOT** a replacement for a prevention plan, any support groups, doctors, or any other form of professional help that you have been getting, or need to obtain. Now, it is an excellent resource and guide during the time you are in programs, or during any point in your new, sober life. What this plan **is** at its core is about bringing the life of your dreams to reality, while maintaining your well-being and health.

Keeping that in mind, the next chapter will show you how to combine the lessons you learned in Chapters Four and Five, and also how to review your progress without judgement. You are strong, empowered to succeed, and your efforts will get you there!

GENERAL POINTS FOR REVIEW

- Change is never easy.

- You deserve joy and success. This can only be achieved by forgiving yourself.
- Stagnancy rarely breeds progress.
- Feel and understand the depths of your emotions then take back control.
- Has your past self caused you to place limitations on your present self?
- Action: nothing happens without it, and in its absence there is detriment and imbalance.
- Avoid the cycle of secrecy.
- Your life is a byproduct of the actions you take.
- When you look ahead in life, what do you see?
- How far ahead do your plans go?
- Five years?
- Day by day?
- Having goals gives you back ownership of your time.
- You are building towards a goal: a well balanced, healthy, sober life.

7

IN REVIEW

Do you remember the different aspects of balance we covered? This Spectrum of Balance will come into play quite often as you navigate the sometimes choppy waters of sobriety. Let's take another look across the different variables that play a role in how balanced a life you are leading. As you make your way through the Spectrum, again, it's to review one of the core principles to the maintenance of your healthy direction. Whereas before you may have skimmed the cover, now we'll reopen the "book" and give a more intense look at the Spectrum of Balance and its varied and moving parts.

As we re-explore these different components, do not be afraid to put your thoughts and answers onto paper or document them somewhere. It is important to be able to chart the differences and improvements starting with when you first began your journey. It is important to see balance as both a priority and a necessary tool that will help you in maintaining sobriety.

A very important rule to keep in mind when going through times of review and reflection is to do it without judgement. This may seem like it should go without saying, but self-judgement and guilt are far too prevalent in the life of those in recovery. When you and others on the same path were feeding the addiction, you rarely allowed yourself the chance to feel the brunt of the emotions from the consequences. Once the haze and numbness are gone and you feel the full weight of the fallout, it is far too easy to live a life of self-hatred and derogatory actions. If you are in that vein of thinking, any nostalgia is tainted with a lens of judgement and undue rage. This mindset does not promote growth; more importantly, this mindset can start to erode the progress made up to that point.

As we continue onward, you will be asked to look back at and reflect on the progress you've made. You may feel triggered by this. Prepare yourself and actively withhold being overly harsh with yourself. Do not be afraid to remove yourself from the situation momentarily in order to reestablish an uplifting environment. Always make time for this when you feel it is needed.

Health and Fitness

This is one of the more important VACI's (Vitally Absorbing Creative Interests) because it not only takes time, it also directly correlates to several other elements of the Spectrum. When you first read through the section in Chapter Four, did anything about your lifestyle then stick out to you? What methods or routines have you put into place since then? Remember that no matter how often, or for how long, you exercise, simply putting the effort to working it into your schedule has created that attention to balance.

Spirituality

As this section in Chapter Four explained, the issue of faith and spirituality will differ from person to person, as will the role it will play in your sober life. In the time from then to now, how have your beliefs or faith impacted how you go about your life? Remember that this element does not specifically relate to religion, and in fact can exist without any integration - now or ever - to any creed. Having faith, especially when recovery is involved, is more about believing in *yourself*.

Take some time now and consider a few things, either in your mind or on paper. How did you feel when you first addressed this issue when it was brought up in Chapter Four? No matter the positive or negative feelings related to that moment, it is important to recall. Now, consider where your faith is in your progress, your life, and your choices. Has it strengthened? If so, where have you seen the most growth. In what circles of your life has it made an impact?

All these questions, and any more that arise during the time taken to give it thought, will enable you to take a step back and view the larger picture. Without belief in the path you are on, without belief in yourself, you cannot be fully set up for success in a life of recovery.

Social Life

Too often this subject matter is put in a negative light when it comes up in review, or at best is viewed with sad nostalgia. While the unfortunate truth, as we discussed earlier, means that ties had to be cut socially when you decided to enter recovery, that is rarely unavoidable. It does not, however, define your entire social identity, especially now as you continue to progress and grow as a person.

Rather than thinking back over what you lost, consider it from a different perspective. What people comprise your support system? It is worth the time to write their names down. By doing this you are putting power behind your gratitude and recognizing those who helped you get to where you are through their efforts and belief. Look through the list you just made and really *see* the people you accounted for. In what ways did they positively impact your journey on an individual, personal level?

Your path here has taken social sacrifices, and those sacrifices were meaningful to you and as such will leave an imprint. During your time from then to now, and truly your recovery as a whole, you have no doubt let your mind think of those you had to distance yourself from. It is for this reason that you are replacing those feelings of nostalgia with the positive power of naming your support group.

Keep that list close and in times when you are lacking confidence or the road seems particularly rough, you can remember that you are loved. The concept of "being loved" can often seem off-hand and emotionless without an anchor in reality, and seeing the names of people in text is proof that this love isn't just an idea, it's a reality.

Romantic Life

Depending on where you are in your recovery, you may or may not be in a place where you are considering adding a romantic element to your life. Programs differ, as do personal preferences, so make sure that is all taken into account when this subject matter is brought up. There is never a rush to form romantic attachments, nor should there be any pressure. As you know by now, any rush will create an imbalance and is not worth jeopardizing your sobriety.

Where are you at this point? If you are still leading up to a point where you will allow yourself that chance, what plan do you have in mind for handling that situation? There should be an expectation of difficulty. Not just in the relationship, but in how it relates to your recovery. The road of recovery is one that lasts for the remainder of your life, as you know, and a romantic interest will impact and be impacted by your life.

On the other hand, you may be well into your sobriety and romance is already incorporated and an important aspect of your life. If this is the case, how does it affect your day-to-day experience? Whether you are in a relationship or not, including the possibility for both attraction and involvement, your sobriety will and must play a role. You lead a life of transparency, and in that spirit any partner you consider including in your life needs to be allowed the chance to consider how it will impact *their* lives as well.

Write out how you view romance, either out loud or on paper to give it power and how you've acted on it. Look at this from three different stages: when you began your sobriety journey; when we discussed it first in Chapter 4; and where you are now. This will let you examine how you've grown, and how your views of romance have either changed or remained steadfast. Love is a vital component of life, and will be a part of yours in some way. Without being able to see how this aspect has been viewed on your journey, you cannot appreciate it and be prepared to take on the responsibility.

Hobbies

While this element of balance can seem simple, it is just as important as the other aspects. Stagnant time is the enemy of sobriety, and as we learned earlier, simply *having* a hobby gives you an outlet when faced with time that has the potential to be unused. When you began this book, did you have any particular hobbies you had taken an interest in? Do you still participate in them, and if not, why did that end? Sometimes activities and other interests are in our life only for a short time, and then they have served their purpose. This is not a negative way to conduct both yourself and how you use your time. Allow yourself the freedom to alter what you put your time and effort into. Your life is centered around your sobriety, and from that will come a great relearning of various habits and patterns. Without the flexibility to adjust along with those changes, you will create unneeded friction in a process that is challenging as it is without any help.

What new activities are a part of your life now? Big or small, it is simply their presence that can matter. If you stopped some hobbies, take a look at why that happened and how you grew from them. As you review these areas, take the time to see how these hobbies and interests impact your schedule. Sometimes you may not realize you are spread too thin until you see it laid out in front of you. If you haven't felt stressed from these activities, chances are you have planned the time well, but it is always worth checking on. Consider it a form of allowing for self-correcting.

Career

The decision to begin a life of sobriety has had an impact across all areas of your life, but there are often more severe or direct consequences in several key areas. Your family and friends are one, and another primary element is how your work, your career, has been, and will be, affected.

Imagine that you had to make a progress chart that showed your job performance. You would plot key moments during your addiction, immediately following your decision of recovery, up until it was directly referenced in Chapter Four, and then now. How would that line's movements look? Where are the peaks and low points? If you feel so inclined, go ahead and sketch out a graph like this. See if you can really think back and calculate the ups and downs so they're plotted into an image. Make it as simple or as detailed as you would like; the goal is to give you a good idea of the progress as a whole.

Once you have done this, and hopefully have had a little "art class" fun while doing it, let's examine the results. Look at the particularly high points; to what real life events do they correlate? Do the same with the areas that are at the lowest. What patterns do you see? How have you made progress within those segments of time laid out before? Perhaps you will notice that you actually need to examine why there isn't more upward movement to where you are now.

The point is to take stock of where you may need to make adjustments, or perhaps to show that you are making the correct steps to ensure your sober life continues. Career can be where you suffered most because of your addiction, and can be the most difficult area to remedy as one in recovery. Do not feel discouraged, regardless of what you find in review; you are making great strides, and the benefits will pay off in their own time.

This may have been the first time you did an in-depth check on how the full spectrum of balance was holding up. Like anything that is a priority, it requires attention and maintenance as time goes on. None of the decisions and practices you are putting into action are single-use, end-all solutions. They are methods and steps along the way. It is important to go back and do these kinds of reviews to ensure you are living a balanced life, because in the hectic, fast-paced world we all must exist in, it can be far too easy to lose track of where the imbalance may be.

Keep the notes and points you made during this self-check so whenever you go through the Spectrum in the future you can refer back. There is a difference between *knowing* you are making progress, and *seeing* the progress you are making. Keeping this kind of information on paper or electronically will prove invaluable later on. Having a visible record will help you create goals and desires to work towards, with concrete reasoning behind them.

Every lesson and guideline you have learned and implemented during this process has all been for a singular goal: to create a balanced system to cultivate your sober life. Every piece is a necessary component to form a lifestyle that is designed to not miss out on any of the richness you can experience. This approach can be referred to as the "never a dull moment" method, or more simply, ways to keep yourself busy, but sober.[1]

A commonly agreed upon truth is that free time is rarely a positive element to occur during the sober routine. This is not saying that your immediate response to having that time will be rushing back to the addiction, but it *does* open the door for thoughts that could very well lead down that road. Until you are more grounded and have proven over time - to yourself and to your life - that you are able to handle those quiet moments, you are susceptible to unhealthy patterns of thought. Guilty ruminations and "what if's" can let doubt seep in, undoing the great work you've done on your confidence and willpower. While it may seem like a harmless event, it is not worth the risk to allow that kind of thinking to take hold.

New habits are difficult to implement, and for the first 30-60 days is a fragile thing indeed. Nearly everything you put into place when starting out on a path of sobriety *is a new habit*. Everything is going to begin from a very fragile place, and will need an added modicum of protection. This protection comes in the form of "time usage." While it is true that there are times when simply "keeping busy" won't be enough, but for the odd times when those empty slots do occur, you'll know how to react.

This process can be a slippery slope to navigate, because while you try to avoid those free times, it is also a necessity to include rest and downtime for yourself. Early on it can be a fine line between the two, and the process should be treated with focus and respect. Where are those places in your life that sparked difficulty early in your journey? How did you respond? Always being on guard and at the ready can be tiring, but it is a necessary challenge for that time. It is for these reasons that having a support system - and leaning on them when needed - is absolutely crucial to succeeding in this new lifestyle.

How are you making time for rest *and* ensuring that time isn't simply empty space that your mind can fill with unnecessary thoughts? This answer will be different for everyone, depending on situations and schedules, but the foundation needs to remain the same: doing everything actively and with awareness. That is how you navigate those sometimes murky waters of knowing when to let go and rest, and when to recognize the time as a negative atmosphere, and responding accordingly.

Maintaining a sober lifestyle is a never-ending pursuit. Day-to-day efforts and beyond, it is a challenge, but remember that it is a challenge you are certainly up for! Aim for success and sobriety and you will be able to follow through with the tools and methods you have learned here. Never stop moving forward with determination and a focus on your goals. Your addiction will always be waiting for you to come back, so you must remain actively aware for the sake of your health and well being. You are *worthwhile* and from that you can find the strength and purpose to persevere when the days seem too long, or the stresses are taking their toll.

Remain steadfast in your avoidance of boredom or idle time that could lead back down paths of negativity and destructive tendencies. You have worked too hard for these emotional pitfalls to ensnare you; take strength and courage from the tools provided in these lessons. You have a purpose, one that you may have lost sight of for a time, but now on this new, fresh road, you can set your sights back on those destinations.

Because of the work you do every day without fail, you have created the framework that can be utilized from here on out. You are empowered to say *no* when you feel a situation will not serve your best interests. The sacrifices made to form a healthy environment will give you the backbone, the power, to make those difficult decisions. Nothing is impossible when your mind and body are working in harmony. Nothing is impossible when you are moving forward towards a brighter horizon with patience and grace. The troubles of your past can be left behind for good and you can feel the freedom to progress in a life without limitations.

You are capable!

You are strong!

You will find your way to lift the weight of addiction.

GENERAL POINTS FOR REVIEW

- Do you remember the Spectrum of Balance?

- As we re-explore these aspects, are you recording your thoughts somewhere?
- Journaling?
- Digitally?
- Voice recording?
- Health and Fitness
- What changes have you made?
- What habits have you put into place?
- Spirituality
- How has belief impacted your life and sobriety?
- This is not necessarily religious belief, but rather a belief in *yourself*
- Social Life
- Whose names are on your list of supporters?
- In what ways did those individuals positively impact your journey?
- You are loved.
- Romantic Life
- Where are you at this point?
- What plans do you have for handling this aspect?
- How does it/will it affect your day to day life?
- Are you living a life of transparency?
- Hobbies
- What hobbies did you have when you began this journey?
- What hobbies do you have now?
- In what forms are they helping you self-correct?
- Career
- What does your progress chart look like?
- Did this give you an idea about your progress as a whole?
- What patterns did you notice?
- Have you made progress in those areas?
- Free time is rarely a positive element to introduce to a sober routine.

- Nearly everything you put into place when starting out on a path of sobriety is a *new habit*.
- Where are the places in your life that sparked difficulty early in your journey?
- How did you respond?
- How are you making time for rest?
- You are empowered to say *NO* when you feel a situation will not serve your best interests.
- *YOU* are capable!
- *YOU* are strong!
- *YOU* will find a way to lift the weight of addiction.

8

CONCLUSION

In this book, you learned how to balance your life, what triggers to identify, and how to live a sober life without judgement. You were challenged and asked to unearth depths of yourself that had been locked up for years, possibly longer. From the beginning, it was stated that by following the steps and lessons along the way you would find purpose, discover new positive characteristics about yourself, and how to live a life free from the weight of addiction. Standing where you are now, I have no doubt you are the living proof of all those elements!

There are few things in this life as difficult as finding the resolve and strength to battle your way out of addiction's grasp. Like many before you, and the many that will follow, you have accomplished something truly incredible. At one point, or several, there may have been no hope, no light, and no love. Yet now, in a new place, you are well on your way to being back in the brightness of sobriety: with hope, in the light, and truly loved.

Here is where our paths part, but in no way are you ever alone. Look to those you love in times when your strength doesn't feel like it's enough. Look inside yourself and find belief in the amazing places you will go and the incredible things you have yet to do! There are not enough words to define the bravery in a life saved by recovery. No one understands that bravery better than you do. You should be very proud of yourself, and every single day from here on out, you deserve to be reminded of that fact.

Thank yourself for this opportunity, and I also thank you for having the power to take control of your life. Addiction is one of the most difficult things in this world to overcome, and you have done that and so much more! Keep taking each step with power and confidence, because you are a being of joy, truth, and strength. Never forget that.

Thank you.

REFERENCES

1. WHAT IS ADDICTION?

1. https://www.verywellmind.com/willpower-101-the-psychology-of-self-control-2795041
2. https://www.ncbi.nlm.nih.gov/pmc/articles/PMC5068365/
3. https://www.ncbi.nlm.nih.gov/pmc/articles/PMC5068365/#ref-39

2. HOW ADDICTION HAPPENS

1. https://www.psychologytoday.com/us/blog/shame/201305/the-difference-between-guilt-and-shame

4. A BALANCED AND PURPOSEFUL LIFE IS A SOBER LIFE

1. https://www.smartrecovery.org/vaci-3/
2. https://www.smartrecovery.org/benefits-of-exercise-in-addiction-recovery/
3. https://castlecraig.co.uk/blog/2019/05/07/7-best-exercises-for-addiction-recovery
4. https://castlecraig.co.uk/blog/2019/05/07/7-best-exercises-for-addiction-recovery
5. https://www.rtor.org/2019/08/12/sobriety-spirituality-and-mental-health/
6. https://www.psychologytoday.com/us/blog/all-about-addiction/201805/7-spiritual-elements-critical-addiction-recovery
7. https://www.hipsobriety.com/home/2014/11/11/sobriety-your-social-life-the-8-things-i-wish-i-had-known
8. https://www.evergreendrugrehab.com/blog/love-sex-and-relationships-in-recovery/
9. https://www.ashwoodrecovery.com/blog/guide-to-relationships-after-addiction/

5. DEVELOPING NEW HABITS

1. https://alcoholrehab.com/addiction-recovery/bad-habits-in-recovery/
2. https://alcoholrehab.com/addiction-recovery/bad-habits-in-recovery/
3. https://www.mindful.org/meditation/mindfulness-getting-started/
4. https://www.floridarehab.com/treatment/addiction-therapies/habit-reversal-therapy/

5. https://baartprograms.com/about-baart/
6. https://baartprograms.com/5-healthy-living-habits-during-recovery/

7. IN REVIEW

1. https://lakehouserecoverycenter.com/blog/keep-yourself-busy-to-keep-yourself-sober/

www.ingramcontent.com/pod-product-compliance
Lightning Source LLC
Chambersburg PA
CBHW022010120526
44592CB00034B/771